Long Shot

Long Shot

MY BIPOLAR LIFE
and the Horses Who Saved Me

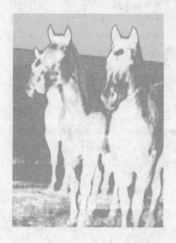

SYLVIA HARRIS

with Eunetta T. Boone and Bill Boulware

ecco

An Imprint of HarperCollinsPublishers

HarperCollins books may be purchased for educational, business, or sales promotional use. For information please write: Special Markets Department, HarperCollins Publishers, 10 East 53rd Street, New York, NY 10022.

A hardcover edition of this book was published in 2011 by Ecco, an imprint of HarperCollins Publishers.

FIRST ECCO PAPERBACK EDITION PUBLISHED 2012.

Designed by Kathryn Parise

Library of Congress Cataloging-in-Publication Data has been applied for.

ISBN 978-0-06-171441-2

12 13 14 15 16 OV/RRD 10 9 8 7 6 5 4 3 2 1

ONE DAY
All the flowers that I've picked . . .
all the shells from the sea . . .
can never ever equal the love you gave to me.

Now as I stand upon this empty shore . . .
I'm wishing for your arms . . .
they can't hold me anymore.

All the scrapes and bruises . . .
the long teary nights . . .
you comforted and guided me . . .
taught me . . . made me . . . stand up and fight . . .

Now you can rest your tired and weary soul.
Your spirit soars with the sky . . .
you have stars to hold . . .
When the wind whispers, and the moon guides my way . . .
I'll fall to my knees asking your Angel wings . . .
to lift me up . . . be with you . . . and pray . . .
Together again . . . ONE DAY.

Contents

✤

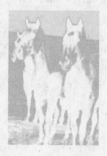

Contents

Preface

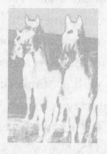

I am small in stature, barely an inch above five feet. But I can put up a good fight, something I've been doing all my life, often with family, friends, and strangers but mostly with myself. I am bipolar and have struggled with it since it surfaced shortly after high school. I ascend to heights of frenetic energy and confidence only to plummet to hellish depths of madness, guided by unseen voices and terrifying hallucinations. Imagine you're watching a DVD or a video, and you pick up the remote and punch fast-forward. Suddenly, those images flash by in milliseconds. The "screen" of my mind operates in the same fashion. It is in manic phase when I sketch voluminous drawings of people, places, horses. And I'll sketch them on anything: paper, napkins, walls, wherever I can create. If I'm not sketching, I'm writing volumes and volumes of poetry or prose with unchained thoughts in my journal, until finally I crash into days of sleep. It is exhilarating while in it, but exhausting coming out of it. More than once I've found myself within the confines of mental institutions, and many more times I've gone off the deep end after tottering on the edge of reality and fantasy, unable to maintain my balance against a whirlwind of raging emotions.

I'm forty-three years old, but my life feels twice that. People say I am an angry woman. I am. When you've had to fight through so many things, it's hard not to be. I have been hungry, cold, abused physically, tormented emotionally, homeless, and frequently out of control. But I've also, at times, lived a seemingly quite normal life with my three children and their father. And against all odds, at forty years old, I became the first African American woman in Chicago racing history to win a race and only the second in U.S. history.

I continue to struggle with being bipolar and always will. But psychotropic medicines, which have not always been available to me, spiritualism, which in my case happens to be Buddhism, and—most important—my love of horses keep me from looking at life as one continuous battle. My life has been a race to outrun the disease that attempts to consume me. To that point, I tell my story in parallel to my biggest race, that cold day in December 2007.

I haven't always been able to live life on my terms, but I'm optimistic I'll get there—even if it is a long shot.

Sylvia Harris
July 2010

The Race

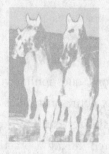

I n an empty stall, at a makeshift altar, I close my eyes and begin my Buddhist chant, *Nam-myoho-renge-kyo*: "Devotion to the teaching of the mystic law of the universe," or even more loosely translated, "Devotion to cause and effect." I chant to quiet my mind in a way that lithium or Haldol cannot. Then I get dressed and head to the paddock.

December in Chicago is brutal. On this snowy Thursday evening, a cold front from Canada is blowing snow and ice into the city, creating dangerous conditions. As I pass through the backstretch, also known as the backside, an area of stables and living quarters for the people who call the track home, little ice pellets stab me in the face, but I don't really feel it. My mind is on Peg. We have a lot in common, Peg and me: a broken horse and his broken rider. He was sired by Fusaichi Pegasus, who won the Kentucky Derby in 2000, a promising mount that never materialized, and I was the all-American girl from Santa Rosa who had long ago lost her way.

Wildwood Pegasus is a four-year-old gelding who has lost his spirit, but I understand him. When you spend time in and out of mental institutions, questioning your reality and making a mess out of your life, your spirit takes a beating that no anti-depressant or mood stabilizer can fix. Pegasus is arthritic, with a bum right leg shattered during a practice run when he was a promising two-year-old. Together, we are a bad bet. Entertaining, maybe, but a bad bet nonetheless.

When I reach the paddock, he is waiting for me. Jockeys can be superstitious. Many have rituals before or after every race. British jockey Graham Thorner wore the same underwear for every race he won after winning the Grand National in 1972. They got so old and frayed that he would wear a new pair over the old ones until he ended his career. Garrett Gomez, one of horse racing's biggest prizewinners, makes sure he steps out of bed with his right foot first on race day; and top jockey Ramon Dominguez reads a quote from Booker T. Washington that's taped to his locker before every race: "Success is to be measured not so much by the position that one has reached in life as by the obstacles which he has overcome." Me, I have two rituals. I chant, and then, before I mount the horse, *I breathe him in.* I know it sounds a little *Horse Whisperer*-ish, but when I breathe in a horse, it's as if we are kindred souls. We are one.

I hold Peg's face in my hands and press my own to his, to breathe my baby in. So there we are, Peg and me, nose to nose; soul to soul. "Peg, my beautiful Peg," I said. "Tonight, it's you . . . you show me. I'm just along for the ride."

I gulp down the freezing air near the paddock as both of Peg's trainers, Charlie and Janelle, come over. Their bright, sunny smiles greet me, and suddenly everything is more than fine. The three of us stand in the cold with a light snow falling and with that beautiful smell of horses filling our noses. We have been working with Peg for weeks, and we instinctively know this is his time. Charlie and Janelle both give me a leg up onto Peg, who waits patiently for us to finish. Once my body connects with his, there is only one way to go. As Peg carries me, I feel as if it's a new day and a new life. I always feel that way when I get on the back of a horse.

Following tradition, we are led to the starting gate by the outrider, Jerry. Life on the backstretch is full of irony. Jerry, an ex-cop with a questionable past, is quite the horseman. Fit and good-looking, he has a deep love affair with cognac, and a few days before we'd had a heated argument in the parking lot of a bar near the track. I don't even remember what it was about, most likely something petty, personal—that's the way it can be on the backstretch, the world behind the racetrack. It's a carnival-like atmosphere filled with runaways, addicts, desperate lost souls, and the rich people who employ them. But when it's time to compete, everyone does his job. Jerry is no different. He throws me a look that says, *Go, Sylvia.* I nod to acknowledge it.

Once we're near the starting gate, I look up to the grand-stand briefly to find my family. They're here visiting me, and for the first time, they will see me ride. I peruse the crowd until I see them looking down at me, wearing mixed looks of pride and concern. They're like many American families, a cornucopia of dysfunction. My father, Edward Sr., a tough ex-army staff sergeant and recovering alcoholic; my mother, Evaliene, an ex-teacher with Crohn's disease who for years was a punching bag for my dad; my brother Edward Jr., the minister—let's just say he's the good one; my oldest children, daughter Shauna and son Ryan, from my common-law marriage with Riley, an Irish hippie I met at a club. And then there was Mioshi, my youngest, the baby who was conceived during a manic farewell tryst in Los Angeles. They were all there together, and for once it was not a gathering to decide, What are we going to do about Sylvia? A rare occasion.

The weather is changing for the worse, and I can feel the icy sleet pounding my face. I know Peg can feel it too. The track will be treacherous, but it is also perfect for Peg's old, worn body, where the soft powder of the snow is like a natural cushion for his knee and ailing bones. Finally, someone or something is delivering him the break he so richly deserves.

This is our second outing together. We came in third a month earlier, and with each workout we began to respect each other more. Despite that, on the backstretch, we are seen as lost causes—me because of my age and inexperience, and Pegasus because he had been winless in his last seven starts. Still, he is more than ready. Me? I'm terrified.

Just a few days earlier, three horses went down on the track with their jockeys in tow. The thought of a half-ton bay horse crashing onto my small frame is scary enough. But what is even more frightening to me is the possibility that a manic episode could happen right before or during the race. Skipping your medications is a big no-no in the bipolar world. The meds are supposed to keep me balanced. But in the horse racing world, a jockey can't take any medications that give him, or her, an advantage.

I'm sure there's an exception for a manic-depressive like me, but I don't want anyone to feel I have to take something that gives me an adrenaline boost. I don't think I've ever been manic while racing, but the exuberant feel of riding gives me the same rush. Normally, I would welcome that feeling of superhuman superiority, but not on race day. It's too dangerous; the chance of losing your focus or miscalculating is too great. This is definitely not the state you want to be in while riding a horse. But when they load me and Pegasus into the gate, I'm normal, or as normal as a nonmedicated manic-depressive can be.

I'm a forty-year-old rookie jockey who's riding her seventeenth race and has never won. I'm a mother deemed unfit by some to raise her own kids. I've been homeless, sleeping in a Jeep, wondering where my next meal will come from.

I am bipolar. And I'm about to win this race.

The Start

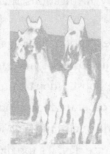

*A*top this thousand-pound mass of horse sits my taut five-foot-one, hundred-and-ten-pound frame. I contrast with the other jockeys in almost every way; my age, my gender, my race. What we all share is a determination to win, but for me this a big race—actually, at my age every race is a big race, but today my family will be looking on, and I so want to show them I can do this, give them something to celebrate instead of the trouble I have been.

Pegasus and I approach the gate, and my nerves do a jig on my body. I breathe faster than Peg can ever hope to run. He seems calm, although he shows some trepidation about entering the gate. I hope this is not a bad sign. Jerry, the outrider, comes over to help guide us into our post position.

The horses are in place. We jockeys are raised a few inches above our saddles with knees tucked in tight, which reduces wind resistance and allows us to lessen the load on our mounts. The grandstands are far from full, but that doesn't change the excitement I feel. The air bristles with sounds, scents, and kinetic

energy. I take it all in, then quiet it to a hush, slowing my sensa-
tions down to a point where I can move easily. Both Pegasus and
I have traveled a long way to run this race. It's a big moment for
both of us.

The gate bell splinters the frozen air.

The horses bolt out of the gate, along with my adrenaline, as
the announcer's voice shouts, "And they're off!"

Santa Rosa, California

"Come on, Daddy, tell me, tell me," I beg him as he drives our
wood-paneled station wagon down a dusty road I do not recognize. I'm twelve years old, and it is a typically sunny day in
Santa Rosa, California, where my family lives. We moved to this
small city, about an hour and a half outside of San Francisco,
once my father retired from the army. Both my parents had
made a career of the military, and with my father's pension and
the job he had at a nearby shipyard, we had enough money for
a nice middle-class life in a comfortable suburban home.

"Tell you what?" he says, feigning innocence, knowing perfectly well what I want. The surprise is the whole reason for
this trip.

"Just give me a hint, *please*," I say, hoping to wear him down.
I know it won't happen, but I enjoy the game.

"If I tell you, that will spoil the surprise."

"No. No way!"

"Okay, then, once I remember what it is, I'll let you know."

I poke him in the arm, then pretend to sulk, which only makes him laugh as I see what appears to be a farm come into view. My mind races to an image that I immediately let go of out of fear of being disappointed. I am silent—still, as if any expression on my part will somehow make it all disappear.

We stop in front of a large barn where a man dressed like a cowboy greets my father. They talk briefly; my father points toward me, then motions for me to join them. I quickly exit the car. My father introduces me as his daughter, and we all three walk past the barn to a corral that holds a beautiful horse. I long to hear the words "He's yours," but I'm too nervous to ask.

I've always loved animals, even the days before we moved to Santa Rosa. Living on different army bases, I would constantly seek the companionship of all types of creatures: snakes, bugs, stray dogs and cats. But there was always something about horses that dazzled me. As a little girl, my father took me on pony rides at local carnivals. Then, when I was around six or seven, he decided we should ride on some "real horses." Plopping me on an adult-size thousand-pound horse, then mounting his own horse, my father rode alongside me. It was the perfect Kodak moment, until suddenly my horse jolted and took off like a shot. My father did his best to follow, but not being that much of a rider, he couldn't keep up.

Flying across a grassy field and hanging on for dear life, I didn't cry. I loosened my grip on the reins and instinctively clenched harder with my thighs; then, and to this day I don't know why, I let go and stretched my arms out to the side as if they were wings. I felt like an angel flying through the clouds. I never felt safer, or more free, than at that moment.

When my father caught up to me, he was amazed that I was so calm. "How did you do that, Sylvia?" I guess he meant, how had I managed to stay on the horse without falling. All I could do was shrug.

"You're a natural, I guess," he said, but still, he took the reins and led us back to the stables.

Since then my father and I had talked about horses, but after my mother scolded him for putting a little girl on a "wild" horse, I thought it could never be more than talk. Yet here we are, standing outside a fence looking at a horse who is looking at us.

We stand there, silently admiring the horse, who moves closer to make sure he has our attention. The suspense is killing me: Why are we here? I look at my father, who just smiles and intentionally looks away. I look back at the horse, who is now snorting, his head bobbing up and down. Is he trying to tell me something? I wonder.

Finally, the man who looks like a cowboy says to my father, "You going to let her know?" I quickly look toward my dad. He seems to be mulling it over. I can take it no longer.

"Daddy! Is he for me?"

"Hmm. Could be."

"Stop teasing her," said the cowboy, "and let her get up on her very own horse."

I scream and hug my daddy. "Thank you, thank you, Daddy. What's his name?"

"Laredo," replied the cowboy. "He's a quarter horse." I didn't care what he was; I just knew he was mine.

For the next few months, I couldn't wait for each school day to end so I could bike to a stable not too far away and bond with my Laredo. I was sure he spent all day just waiting for me to show up and tell him all about my boring day at school. It didn't hurt that I sometimes would bring carrots for him.

One day I raced to the stable, as usual, only to find that Laredo was gone. No one at the stables had an answer for me, so I biked home as fast as I could. I found my mother cooking dinner and begged her to tell me what had happened to Laredo. She wouldn't talk about it, and told me to speak to Dad. I discovered my father had sold Laredo. It was too expensive to take care of him. My father suddenly needed the money, which I couldn't understand. After all, my family was living the American dream on a quiet cul-de-sac in Santa Rosa. I took piano and dance lessons and went water skiing. I thought if we just got rid of all of those lessons, there would be more than enough money to take care of Laredo. I begged my father to get Laredo back, but he turned a deaf ear.

"Horses aren't important," he told me. "Go do your school-work and stop bothering me about this nonsense."

I went to my mother, hoping she might influence my dad. "Can't you get Daddy to change his mind? Please, Mom. I won't need any Christmas or birthday presents—ever," I said.

"Your father knows best, Sylvia," which was code for they weren't speaking. I may have only been twelve turning thirteen, but I knew my parents barely talked to each other. There always seemed to be something going on between them. My mother was little, like me, and hadn't been healthy for years. She had Crohn's disease, a chronic, episodic, inflammatory bowel disease that at times caused her great pain and forced her to undergo several surgeries. At one point, she even went down to seventy pounds and couldn't lift herself out of the bed. My baby brother and I would try to help, but most of the load fell to my father, and he seemed to resent it.

There was nothing left for me to do about losing my horse but to cry on the shoulder of my best friend, Gidget. Yes, that was really her name—Gidget Harding—and she lived across the street from me. Where I lived was truly a slice of American idealism. And even though we were the only African American family around, everyone was friendly and supportive and race never seemed to be a factor. Not only did I cry on Gidget's shoulder but also on her lavender-flowered bedspread and the teen magazines she tried to show me to get my mind off of losing Laredo. Before long she was crying too, and we consoled each other by promising to one day get our own horses. We then calmed down and began to think of names for the horses we would have one day.

"Alice," she suddenly blurted out.

I told her that was kind of a plain name for a horse.

"No," she said. "I'm talking about Alice Patterson. She lives on a farm. They must have horses. Maybe she'll let us ride them."

My excitement over this idea brushed away the sadness I was feeling, and we immediately called Alice. The next few months I consoled myself with visits to Alice's farm, where there were beautiful working horses. The three of us were like Charlie's Angels on horseback. We would ride bareback through the farmlands by her house. "I'm sliding off! I'm sliding off!" I would cry, but I never did. Riding always came naturally to me.

It was only a few times that we got to ride the horses at Alice's. They were needed for other duties. Eventually, my parents tired of me hounding them about another horse. To divert my pleading, they made me take ice-skating, piano, and dance lessons. I enjoyed the diversions, but I never stopped longing for a horse.

I was always athletic and enjoyed sports. I became quite the star in gymnastics and track, winning meets and even participating in the state championships. The competition and success I had helped to distract me from the growing tension between my parents. The strain of my mother's illness and her needs were taking a toll on their relationship. Always a heavy drinker, my father began to indulge more and more. Violent arguments between my parents soon became standard fare.

"Did you fall and get those bruises, Evaliene?" he would ask innocently the next morning while she cooked him breakfast. She'd nod dutifully and serve up his bacon and eggs. I sort of knew what was going on but never fully acknowledged it, preferring a loose sort of denial. As an adult, I now know that when he hit my mother, he was in an alcoholic blackout, but as a child it threw me. Not just his questions about what had happened, but the way these periodic outbursts—coming after days of binge drinking—contrasted with the life we projected to those around us . . . just a normal middle-class family.

We made the most of the natural splendor unique to Northern California. We would escape to the local parks and lakes for waterskiing or camping. It was hard for my mother to travel with us when she was ill, but somehow the four of us would drive to Lake Tahoe for mini holidays. On those vacations, as we sat at restaurants, we seemed like a regular, normal family enjoying each other's company. For a few days, we would play the roles of loving husband, father, daughter, and son. But there were still few signs of affection between Mom and Dad. I rarely saw them holding hands, and hugs were not the norm for any of us.

I liked school but became a bit of a loner. Except for class or participating in school activities, like track, I wasn't very outgoing. Even my relationship with Gidget and April waned. I felt more comfortable around my pets—dog, cat, whatever creature I might be befriending at the time—than around other kids. My place of choice at home was in my room, reading or doing experiments with my chemistry kit.

All that came to an abrupt halt when I turned sixteen.

I decided to ditch the quiet Sylvia and became a cheerleader. Blame my hormones—I was no different from the other girls who were really getting into boys and the requisite trouble that often follows those first brushes of freedom and young love. I'd sneak alcohol out of the cabinet and join some of my fellow cheerleaders at one of their homes that would be parent-free for most of the night. We'd put on some loud Pat Benatar music and have our version of a wild evening. As Pat crooned, "Hit me with your best shot," I even tried my first hits of pot, but back then I wasn't a big fan of drugs. It only made me sleepy.

My drug of choice was going to the Bay Meadows Golden Gate Fields with my father when the horses were racing. I'd sit in those metal stands and feel the thunder and the power of the Thoroughbred racehorses. I was a runner and they were runners, so I identified with their every step. With my mouth wide open, I'd watch them sail through the air and silently wish I could be their rider so I could feel weightless and free.

I kept up the partying for the rest of high school, getting smashed on alcohol just about every weekend. My parents would give me the occasional lecture, and a couple of times I got in trouble for leaving without telling them; I would just look them in the face and lie.

"I didn't do it," I'd say in my most casual of voices. "I was home the entire time."

"Sylvia, I checked your bedroom. You were gone," my mother said.

"I was in the other room," I'd fib with a straight face, and most of the time my mother would just sigh and give up. She was too sick to really delve into my problems, and my parents remained on extreme edge with each other, which left them little time for dealing with adolescent concerns. Eventually, I got the attention I thought I deserved from a pretty serious boyfriend who was the handsome, charismatic star football player at the rival school in town.

Broad-shouldered and sweet, Dan was a year ahead of me, and when he graduated, he signed up for the marines. We had the summer together before he had to take off. The night before he left, he took me in his arms. "Wait for me, Sylvia," he pleaded.

I promised that I would, if we could get married and start our own family. The idea of my own home and a husband seemed blissful to me; I could leave the escalating baggage behind and be a part of a real family.

Deeply in love and planning my future, I'd run to the mailbox each day for his daily letter from boot camp, and I missed him in the way you only can with a first love. That fall, my senior year, I was nominated for homecoming queen. The one problem was, I didn't have a date because my marine was off at training, and my father flatly refused to escort me.

"I'm busy that night" was all he said. He had grown very distant and tried to spend most of his free time away from us and the house.

My last resort was asking my track coach to take me to the big dance, which was completely humiliating. To top it off, I didn't win the crown; it was first runner-up for me. Without much enthusiasm, I had stepped onto the stage in the school gym to accept my award when my broad-shouldered, handsome ex–football star walked in like something out of a movie. It was my Dan, and now I felt like a winner. Later that night, he asked me to marry him with a beautiful diamond and emerald ring as my prize. He had to go the next day, but he more than made my night. It was enough to get me through the rest of the school year. With a happy new life awaiting me, I even buckled down and focused on my studies.

A few weeks before my high school graduation, my fiancé sent me a thicker letter, and I couldn't wait to rip it open. I thought that maybe he had written me a few poems or enclosed a few drawings, because he liked to sketch in his free time. Instead, he sent a picture of a woman holding a baby. His baby.

Crushed, I didn't get out of bed for the next few days. My mother tried to comfort me, but a bout of her illness was causing her to stay in bed much of the day. Eventually, this made me push aside my own misery and try to help out around the house. Dad was more distant than ever and didn't question or show much concern for us. He would go to work, hang out, sometimes all night, and speak very little when around the house.

Having to help out more got me out of my rut, and I was determined to shake myself free from the sadness and celebrate my graduation. Even if it was not going to lead to the future I had hoped, it was still a new beginning—a fresh start. And in the days that led up to graduation, I joined my classmates in the excitement of our big event.

On graduation day the sky was a brilliant blue, and so was I, in a powder blue dress under my ceremonial black robe, replete with baby blue eye shadow to match the dress. I even had on blue high heels, and I knew I looked good.

After the ceremony, the sun was beating down on everyone, but no one really cared. I saw my father off to the side of the field. It didn't surprise me that he wasn't near my mother, who was sitting in the shade, with my brother fanning her. I walked over to him unsteadily, as my extremely high heels kept sinking into the turf of the football field. I thought at first he was smiling, proud to see his little girl holding her diploma and the many awards I had won for track and field. But once near him, I could see he was only squinting in the sharp sunshine.

"I can't do this anymore," he said as he handed me a graduation card with five hundred dollars in it. He stood there for a moment as if he were going to explain himself, but then he turned and walked away.

"Daddy?"

He didn't stop, and I watched the wrinkled back of his tan suit as he faded away. The next day he packed up his stuff and moved back to Virginia, where we had once lived when I was very young.

What followed were really rough years where my mom was on disability and I felt myself sinking deeper into some sort of emotional abyss. It was a year later that I had my first bipolar episode.

Furlong One

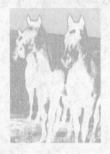

*T*he horses charge out of the starting gate, but Pegasus hesitates slightly. When horses break free they don't all do so equally; sometimes a horse will get off to a quick start. And other times, it may seem somewhat uninterested, as if to say, "No one asked me if I felt like racing today." This seems to be Pegasus's mood, but maybe it's his arthritic knees. I rubbed them frequently before the race, but it's cold today and they could still be stiff. Hopefully, they will begin to warm up. I'm determined not to worry because I know Pegasus would sense my concern and become overly cautious. I have to run my race.

The horses bunch toward an inside position, shortening the length of the track. We are near the back, but for now that's okay. Our time will come.

I no longer hear the announcer or the crowds cheering. All I hear is the roar of hooves pounding the surface of the cold, hard ground. The sounds and motions encapsulate me. The noise is so loud it seems to come from inside my head, but that's okay.

I'm used to hearing all kinds of things in my head. That started long ago.

Santa Rosa, California

For days I had been feeling a strange burst of energy. My mind had been racing with thoughts and ideas, always changing, just enough to register an emotion but too short to contemplate. I would sit in my pink-shag-carpeted room, with its white four-poster bed and matching dresser, and write for hours on end, trying to express these revelations in poetry. Sleep was unnecessary, and I barely ate, yet it all felt somehow natural to me—enjoyable even. Colors, sounds, and images were more vivid and beautiful, as if a layer of thick plastic had been peeled away from my reality. I felt I was having some type of transformation, like Peter Parker in *Spider-Man*. When manic, you believe that whatever is happening is special. That is, until you start doing crazy things, like when I frantically searched for every bit of money I could find in my room and then, under the watchful eyes of my Sean Cassidy, Leif Garrett, and Prince posters, promptly tossed every cent out the window. It felt of the utmost urgency to carry this out. Why? I didn't know, and it didn't matter. I was being swept along by something greater than me. And soon it turned dark. That's how it felt the night the skies opened up and dumped acid rain and frogs onto my street.

I saw my neighbors falling to their lawns in agony, their flesh melting in the torrid acid rain. The scent was overpowering, a foul, blackening smell that gripped my stomach and threatened to slide through my chest and percolate from my mouth. I slammed my bedroom window to shut out the stench and backed away from it, as if that would do any good. I knew the rain would penetrate my house, burning through any place I hoped to hide.

"It's killing everyone in the neighborhood," I screamed. "It's killing all the animals." My mother came into my room, confused and worried, wanting to know what was wrong. I forced her to the window so she could see for herself.

"You see? We have to get out of here. We need to retreat, get everyone from the neighborhood so we can move to another planet. There's only horrible death here for us." And then it started raining frogs; huge green toads that hit the ground, bursting and scattering like water balloons upon contact. "It's too late." I sobbed.

"Sylvia, something is wrong with you. What is it?" I couldn't answer. I felt numb and dropped to my pink shag rug, sitting there withdrawn and lost. My mother called our family doctor, who phoned in a prescription for Valium at a nearby pharmacy. She also called my boyfriend at the time, Tom. He was a big, six-foot-two man in his late twenties who knew how to stay calm in bad situations, a skill he'd learned as a corrections officer. He tried to console me as he scooped me up off the pink shag, took me outside, and put me in his car. My mother got in the back with me, and we drove off.

By the time we got to the drugstore, my terror had morphed into euphoria. I insisted on going inside, where I danced and twirled and sang in the aisles, then pulled down a metal shelf full of seaweed soap. At the time, it was the most important thing in the world. I had to have it. My mom and Tom quickly deduced that a little Valium wasn't going to help. Tom whisked me out of the store, back into the car, and straight to a local hospital, Oakcrest, a facility that specialized in mental illnesses. Once there, the nurses listened to my ramblings. I told them about the "voices" I was hearing, and that I was the messenger for the forthcoming holocaust. I told them I hadn't slept in four days and had been encoding messages to abandon the planet immediately.

The nurses, angels when I look back now, seemed grateful I'd told them of the impending doom. They kept telling me I was tired and needed rest. They gently helped me lie down on a gurney and then gave me a couple of injections that lulled me to sleep. As the nurses left, I heard a loud click as they locked the heavy door. I woke up the next day feeling more like my old self. The doctor at Oakcrest didn't seem overly concerned. He never used the words "mania," "bipolar," or "manic-depressive." His diagnosis: a temporary breakdown because of my father leaving. But it was just the beginning, as I struck out on a path that would take me from sweet little all-American Sylvia to nut-case Sylvia. It was 1986; I was nineteen.

I became a regular at Oakcrest. My problems became a part of my identity. I had been a burgeoning track star, known as the fastest girl in the county; now I was the crazy girl who was caught in the revolving door at Oakcrest. After each hospitalization, I was determined to reclaim my normal life, often working two or three jobs at a time and taking classes to better myself. A person with a mental illness shouldn't be able to do that, right? At least, that's what I told myself. So I enrolled in a beauty college and became an aerobics instructor.

My family had learned how to cope—Dad, by not being around; Mom, by taking me to Oakcrest when I got *weird*. My brother, Edward Jr., just kind of watched the Sylvia show. Poor kid, he didn't know what to do. He didn't talk about it. None of us would talk about it. Somehow, we managed to play "happy family" while living in our own private hell.

Even my best friend Gigi didn't know the extent of my condition; I hadn't told any of my friends what happened that first night I went to Oakcrest. I also never really explained my subsequent visits. If I had to, I would pass it off as a trip to the hospital because of some bug I had caught. I wanted to believe the doctor's diagnosis that it was a passing condition, and because my mother rarely talked about it, I thought it best to be quiet. There was, and still is, a stigma attached to serious mental health problems, and I didn't want to be thought of as a mental case by my friends.

Even now, I'm always in constant fear of not appearing normal. In the beginning, I didn't know how to recognize an oncoming episode. The fear or anger that can be an ordinary response to events can feel like being manic to me too. I can't tell if a burst of creative energy is real or a misfiring in my brain. At times, it's almost impossible for me to tell when I'm manic. The change can be so gradual that the choices I make seem perfectly normal. But the result may be far from it.

This was especially true when, in early 1987, after beginning to feel better—almost normal, I thought—I visited clubs with my girl Gigi. We were two hot girls: Ebony and Ivory. We'd get dressed up and tried to act like a couple of seasoned rocker chicks. This required us to play more mature. When manic, I played it to the hilt.

One night we hit a popular club, and I was feeling a surge of energy. That night the stars seemed brighter, the air crisper. It had been two years since my first episode, and I still wasn't sure what was happening to me as I flowed in and out of moods. But that night I was having fun and feeling pretty, wearing a flower in my hair the way Diana Ross did when she played Billie Holiday in *Lady Sings the Blues*. Toward the end of the night I spotted, across the room, what I knew was my own Billy Dee Williams, except he was Irish, tall and broad-shouldered, with deep, rich green eyes and a long ponytail. He moved with a confidence I found sexy. Immediately, I felt we were destined to be together.

I made my way over to him and asked him to dance. Amused, he agreed. As I led him to the dance floor, my girlfriend whispered, "Watch out. He's trouble." So what, I thought. I'm *crazy*.

He wasn't much of a dancer, but I didn't care. His name was Riley McKnight, and I was hypnotized by those green eyes. That night we made plans to see more of each other, which quickly became a frequent occurrence. For weeks it was heaven. He drove a TR6 convertible, wore the best clothes, always had a roll of bills in his pocket, and took me to the best restaurants from Santa Rosa to San Francisco.

We spent every day and every night together. I loved his house. It was warm and homey. He was a gifted painter, with his own art decorating the walls. His passion was rock and roll, and he was a wannabe musician who didn't quite have the talent. Still, he did his best to be around music, and many of his friends were musicians. They would often come by his house and jam, with Riley shaking a tambourine as he attempted to be a part of the "band."

When he told me all of his secrets, I didn't blink. I had my own secret, which I was hesitant to mention. My bizarre behavior had eventually sent my previous boyfriend Tom packing, and I believed my mother's illness had a lot to do with Dad leaving. It seemed to me that if you're sick and want to keep your man around, the best thing to do is to keep quiet about your illness. So I talked about art and music, asked questions about what Ireland was like. I never told him about my problem.

We were having a wonderful time with weekend trips to San Francisco and Napa Valley. We even went to Hawaii for a week. The weeks together quickly turned into months and despite having my own apartment, I was practically living at Riley's. By the fall, my brother was off to college and, with me hardly ever around, my mother decided to move to Seattle to be near family and friends. It was just Riley and me. My behavior would get erratic at times, but Riley just considered me to be fun-loving and overly energetic; over time, though, it wasn't easy to hide my true condition.

My mania finally showed up during a party one night at Riley's house. His musician friends would come over to buy and smoke weed, then cover the songs of the day. Riley was on a beer run when it happened. I was sitting there, watching the fun. I didn't smoke weed because I was afraid it might trigger an episode. But it might not have mattered that night. I was on a high of my own and had been cycling for days. A tweaking, rising energy kept surging through my body, making me feel as if I were about to burst. Then a voice whispered to me, but there was no one there. It was an invitation, asking me to follow it, and I did. Walking out of the house and into the night, I left the party for one of my own.

When Riley got back, he noticed I was gone. His friends told him I'd been acting really strange. Riley didn't know I had been zooming the last few days; he just thought I was being his fun-loving, high-energy girlfriend. He didn't know that I hadn't slept in days—while he was sleeping, I was up all night, writing poetry and songs of my own. But he knew if I had taken off in the middle of the night without the car, something was wrong.

He found me at the lake near his house. I was naked, walking into the water toward the spaceship I knew was waiting for me at its bottom. I begged Riley to join us. I told him the spaceship had been sent by the voice, who told me to get on it before our planet was destroyed. Instead, Riley managed to talk me into putting my clothes back on. Then we went back to his place, where the party was dwindling down. He took me to the bedroom and got me to lie down. Moving from what I now know was a manic stage to depression, I finally fell asleep.

When I woke up the next morning I told him everything. I watched his facial expression change from one of concern to one that seemed full of panic. I asked him to take me to Oakcrest, but he wasn't having it. He took me to my apartment and told me to rest. I didn't see or hear from him for a week. I assumed he had left, as most people in my life had. But the following week, he called and said he missed me. We picked up right where we left off and were even more intense. I was in love again and our life was good, but I couldn't help feeling like something was different. Even with no episodes or strange behavior from me, Riley watched closely, as if he was waiting for the next disaster to occur.

I had taken an extreme interest in crystals and their so-called mystical auras that were popularly associated with them by many believers of unconventional thought. I began trying to read auras and to use crystals in ways I thought could alter the energy around me. I had taken them with me when Riley arranged for us to take a romantic camping trip. One night he found me away from the cabin, in the woods, spreading my crystals around and meditating over them. I had seen a meteor shower and considered it a sign for me to communicate with a higher energy. Although nothing else happened, Riley was certain I was about to blow. He took me to see a renowned psychiatrist in San Francisco. The doctor didn't diagnose me as bipolar, but after a few sessions he warned the both of us that I would undoubtedly have more episodes, probably for the rest of my life. This was enough for Riley. "I can't do a mental girlfriend," he said. He took me back to my apartment and faded out of my life.

My life quickly turned bleak. I was sick over my separation from Riley and was trying, unsuccessfully, to keep from blaming myself. I was lonely and heartbroken, and I withdrew from my friends out of fear that I might slip into an episode in front of them. And with my rich boyfriend gone, it was difficult for me to make ends meet. It wasn't long before I ended up moving to Seattle to be with my mother.

I worked on getting my license as a certified nurse's aide and also worked a part-time job at Frederick & Nelson, the best department store in Seattle. I was at the Chanel counter, the first black person ever hired in the cosmetics department. I was proud of that. In a short time, I seemed to be getting my life back together. I was handling Mom's bills and mine, and making sure she was getting the proper health care she needed. But there was something else wrong. I was throwing up almost every morning.

A doctor confirmed my worst fear: I was pregnant. There's no way I can do this, I thought. I have to get an abortion. I could've called Riley, but I didn't want to involve him. He'd already dumped me twice because he couldn't handle my illness. I knew he wouldn't be happy about me being a mentally ill mom.

While I struggled with what to do, I was getting bigger by the minute. Every morning I thought, This is the day I'm going to the clinic. But I kept putting it off. By the end of my fourth month, I was resigned to having the baby. But I wasn't sure how I was going to care for it. My mom said with God's help we'd make it through. And then out of the blue, Riley called.

He said that he'd had a dream about me holding a baby girl, and was calling to see how I was doing. I couldn't believe it. How did he know? It had to be a sign. I took a deep breath and spilled the news about the baby. Rather than the harsh response I expected, he told me he would get to Seattle as soon as he could. And boy, did he come through. We started seeing each other again, and before long I was living in an expensive apartment by a shimmering lake. He gave me a credit card to buy whatever I needed and went with me to all my doctor appointments. We even drove up to Canada for a short vacation. I was episode-free, and I thought that despite what the doctor in San Francisco had told us, maybe my disorder was a thing of the past.

Although Riley had to occasionally head back to California to, as he said, take care of his business, he was never gone for long. He was a wonderful expectant father. We were both hippies and decided that we did not want our firstborn to enter the world in such a sterile atmosphere as a hospital. We had her at home. Riley was a great coach as he held my hand when our beautiful daughter, Shauna, was born. Finally, life was good.

It wasn't long before Riley wanted us all to move back to California. He even agreed to get a place for my mother. I couldn't say no. So we moved into a wonderful condo back home in Santa Rosa, at what was a staggering price for that time. But, as Riley told me, "Business is good." I wanted to keep working, but Riley insisted I focus on taking care of the baby. I spent days bonding with Shauna and feeling like I could breathe for the first time in a long while. There were still no signs of my illness, and Riley never mentioned it. It was a wonderful time, until his mother from Ireland—let's just call her Irene—came for an extended stay. Riley wanted Irene to bond with me and her new grandchild, but from the first meeting we immediately did not like each other.

It always amazes me how grandparents can love the grandkids unconditionally but despise the very woman who carried them. She never approved of me and openly expressed concern

that Shauna would become too dark. I used to catch Irene checking Shauna's coloring closely to see if she was going to be dark
like me. She hated me even more when I got pregnant again, six
months after baby Shauna was born. It caught us by surprise. I
felt like I had just adjusted to having one child, and now a second one? Riley shared the same sentiment when I told him. All
he could say was the F-word repeatedly.

"Oh, God, this will ruin my son. Children are so expensive.
And the two of you are not even married. Why are you doing
this to him?" Irene ranted. I used to pray for the day when she
would go back to Ireland. I began to have thoughts of pushing
her over the balcony. I figured I could always claim to be having
one of my episodes. For a while, this thought kept me smiling
and shielded me from her daily verbal attacks. Despite his concerns about a second child, Riley soon became as enthusiastic
about this baby as he had been about Shauna. But his mother
was still a problem.

I hadn't had any episodes in some time, but I began to think
one might come on. I convinced Riley that the stress his mother
was causing me might send me over the edge. To seal it, one
day I casually mentioned to him that I hadn't slept the previous
night and didn't feel the least bit tired. He was familiar enough
with the disorder to know this could be the beginning of a
setback. It wasn't long afterward that Riley put his mother on a
plane back to Ireland.

With Irene gone, I was back to playing happy family with
Riley and Shauna as we waited for the new baby. I had a difficult labor with the birth of my second child. This baby was
larger, and it proved to be quite painful, but when it was all

done, I had the most gorgeous son imaginable. We named him Ryan. Our family was growing, and Riley was rolling in money. He moved us into a bigger house, and made sure the latest cars sat in our driveway. We were happy and we didn't want for anything. The children were always dressed in the cutest clothing and had more toys than they knew what do with. The family became a familiar sight at the local finer restaurants. It was a plush life, and relatively problem-free. But there was trouble brewing: I began to feel the unwanted rustling of my emotional state.

Our relationship became strained as I began to criticize Riley's livelihood, even though it afforded us a very good life. I expressed my desire to do more than be a stay-at-home mom. I decided to return to working part time as a home-nursing assistant. I also got involved with the local theater and started to think about an acting career—something I kept from Riley, knowing he would be critical. Although I enjoyed this change of pace, it only served to increase the tension between the two of us. Riley was not happy about me being away from the house and kids and he let me know it.

Buddhism also began to play a larger role in my life. I had become interested in it before I moved to Seattle, and now I decided to dedicate more time to it. I practiced Nichiren Shoshu, one of many Buddhist denominations that is often described as orthodox Buddhism and in which chanting is an important element of the faith. Although this type of Buddhism is not very common in America, it is practiced by many people around the world.

I found that the community, principles, and chanting helped me survive the stress that was too often in my life. To me, other than being around horses, Nichiren Shoshu is the best prescription for trying to keep myself level. I started chanting twice daily, in the morning and the evening. It helped to calm me as matters deteriorated between Riley and myself. It also gave me the strength to stand up to him. He was growing his business, and I felt those demands did nothing to harmonize our situation. I begged him to slow down for everyone's sake.

We argued more frequently about it, and he began to criticize my interests in everything. It was becoming increasingly clear to me that basing a relationship solely on having kids was like leaving the gas on in an unlit oven; sooner or later there was going to be an explosion.

The underlying stress was building. Sometimes the change can be so gradual, it's like a slow burn from normal to manic. Manic or not, I'd been thinking about moving to Los Angeles, and I felt like the kids needed a change. There were to be auditions with the Pearl Chorus, a renowned international Buddhist choir in Santa Monica. I decided I could sing. I sounded good to myself, and would sing along sometimes when Riley and the boys jammed in our living room. "The Impossible Dream" was my song choice.

One idea spurred another, and before long I had a plan. I would go to Los Angeles to sing in the chorus, get a place, and find a job until I realized my dream of becoming an award-winning actor or singer or both, then send for the kids. I would do it all.

Yeah, I was manic.

Furlong Two

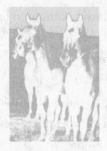

*A*n order is being established as some of the horses accelerate. I feel the urge in Pegasus. He wants to bolt with them. I know he wants to show them who they're dealing with, but I hold him back. It's too early. In a race, it's easy to get ahead of yourself. I know what that can be like. It's characteristic of my illness. I've rushed to places in my head that I was incapable of getting to, where wild, stampeding emotions took control instead of my controlling them. It was not the way to win. As much as I want to run with Peg and let him shine, I know I have to be patient for him. The excitement of the race can burn you out.

I remember words told to me a long time ago by a horseman who had become like a second father to me.

"Have a little bit for now. Have a little bit for later," I softly speak to Peg.

Los Angeles, California

As usual, when I would get what I now know to be manic, my confidence was overflowing. The voices inside of me were clear: "Leave Riley, go to Los Angeles to become a successful actress, then come back for the children." It all made sense to me. The Buddhist choir was a "sign" to get me to Hollywood. It wasn't as if I didn't have any experience; I had performed in a few local theater productions. I was ready for the next step. Weren't you supposed to pursue your dreams? Countless others had, and had succeeded, why not me? I had a gift and was going to Hollywood to share it. And in my spare time, I was going to sing with the internationally acclaimed Buddhist choir the Pearl Chorus.

Never once did it cross my mind that over the years my dreams seemed to be constantly changing. It didn't matter. I was determined. And I just knew it was the perfect way to save my children. Rolling down the I-5 highway, with the windows down and the cold night air washing over me, I imagined the kind of house I would have, right on the beach. The kids and I could play in the sand every day, and we would have lots of pets and maybe a ranch near Santa Barbara where we each would have our own horse. I began naming the horses: Hollywood, the Dream Machine, Superstar.

It was in the wee hours of morning when I pulled into Santa Monica. The city was still. With all of five hundred dollars in my pocket, the best place for me to stay was in my Volvo. I parked in front of the World Cultural Center for Buddhism, and for the next two days that was my hotel. I felt safe there and considered it only temporary. I was a certified nursing assistant; I felt positive that I could find work.

The next morning I signed with a temp agency that soon found me work with AIDS patients. I'd hoped to get a live-in assignment to avoid paying rent, but there wasn't one available. Still, I considered this progress and a positive result of my increased chanting. As a Nichiren Buddhist, I believed strongly in the power of chanting to bring positive results in my life and had increased the number of hours I spent on it. Sure enough, I found an ad for a cheap place to live: it cost $400 a month, which didn't leave me with much else, but at least I would have four walls, instead of a car, surrounding me. I moved in and bought some Campbell's tomato soup. I had to cook it in a partially rusted cookie tin because I couldn't afford to buy pots and pans. It wasn't much, but it was a start.

I was in Los Angeles as the HIV/AIDS epidemic began to peak. One of my first patients lived in a house on Mulholland Drive, a long, twisting road with many spectacular homes that crested the hills between Los Angeles and the San Fernando Valley. On my first visit to Fiona, her front door was open, and I could hear her weeping when I slowly entered the house. She had been stuck in a chair in the kitchen for days, and no one had heard her cries for help. She hadn't eaten or bathed during the entire time. I cleaned her up, got her to eat, and comforted her by holding her, which at the time many people were afraid to do. In fact, the fear of AIDS was more prevalent than the disease itself. Many of these AIDS patients had been at one time vital, successful people who were essentially abandoned and shunned. It was so wrong, and my heart went out to them. I was happy to do all I could for them.

Fiona, who was also a Buddhist, and I became and remained good friends until she passed away.

I got to be friends with Walter, who had been actress Teri Garr's hairstylist. He was a kindhearted man who was deep in the grips of the disease. I would take care of him and even administered his medicine, because the nurses were too afraid of contact to give it to him. More important, I kept him company. Many a night I would crash there after my shift because he didn't want to be alone. I was there for him when even his family turned their backs on him. He was my friend, and I appreciated the companionship as much as he did.

It was rewarding to care for patients who needed me as much as I needed them. But even that wasn't enough to stave off the loneliness I felt without my children. Riley, already upset over this whole situation, was even more sure that my working with AIDS patients was another manifestation of my insanity. I explained to him that I had educated myself on the subject and that with the proper precautions there was no chance of me contracting the disease from my patients. Still, for a while, he considered me to be a risk to the children.

Our talks became nothing but shouting matches, so I decided to focus my attention on the upcoming auditions for the Pearl Chorus. As a practicing Buddhist, I wanted to do that more than anything. I sang day and night. In the shower, in the kitchen, in bed, in the Volvo, anywhere I could. I guess I overdid it. The day of the audition, my voice was gone. Nothing. Nada. When it was my turn to sing, all I could manage was a low squeak. I was more than surprised when the director announced that the newest member of the group would be Sylvia Harris.

My work with the Pearl Chorus was a joyful experience, although it was certainly challenging learning songs in Japanese. But it did little to stop that ever-growing hole in my heart. After about a month, I convinced Riley to let me come to Santa Rosa to see the children on the weekends. It was clear that my being in Los Angeles was devastating for all of us. The children couldn't understand why I had to go back to L.A., and I couldn't get them to understand why I couldn't stay. Nothing had changed between Riley and me. He would just repeat his theory that he shouldn't have to change anything to keep the family together. If that was the case, then my choice was clear.

I would drive back to Los Angeles, and during those lonely hours on the highway, my mind tried to figure out a plan to take the children with me permanently, but there was no easy solution. I couldn't afford to keep them, and I didn't want all of us to go on welfare. All I could do was stick to my plan.

In Los Angeles, work continued to flow in, and I got a job as a live-in cook for a Jewish couple in Hancock Park while still caring for my AIDS patients. The Richbergs were very good to me. They didn't know about my secret, but they knew I practiced Buddhism and were not bothered by my chanting. And they knew that like most young women, so it seemed in Los Angeles, I wanted to be an actress. The wife, Gina, was a retired psychologist, and her husband was a movie executive with a major studio. They both encouraged me as I went on auditions and allowed for a flexible schedule for me to tend to my patients.

Living in Los Angeles agreed with me. It's a city filled with kooks. It's not unusual to see actors dressed as pirates or aliens in studio parking lots reciting lines over and over again, reminding me of some of the people at Oakcrest. But being an actor was more difficult than I had anticipated. Moreover, I didn't have sufficient training, nor the time to get it. I auditioned often with little result. I thought I had a real chance with the sketch show *In Living Color*. I went to an open call and stood in line for five hours to audition for the casting director. When I finally got my turn, I was asked to do a comedic pantomime of my purse being snatched while at a bus stop. I ran around the room, punching and swinging at the air. I'm sure I looked crazy because I felt crazy. And I know crazy. Acting is a lot harder than it looks. I didn't get that part, or any parts, except for a spot in the chorus of a local music production and as an extra for an experimental film. I wasn't having much success as an actress, but I was keeping an even keel even though the marathon debates with Riley about our children were maddening. I wanted the children with me; he wanted them with him.

We weren't exemplary parents back then, Riley and I, but we loved our children, and he knew that my children missed me as much as I missed them. Still, I was surprised when one night he called me while I was in my room at the Richbergs', sounding sweet and nice again. So I suggested, "Why don't you and the kids come for a weekend in L.A.? Let's see if we can all get along."

"Otherwise, what? You're going to sue me for the kids?" a suspicious Riley demanded. I had already decided in my head that I wouldn't use the courts to solve our problems. I would solve everything in my life through faith alone. I concentrated on having a wonderful weekend at Disneyland with Riley and the kids. It was like we were on a family vacation. We went to Disneyland, to the beach, and to the movies. The best times were when we just sat around the hotel room and laughed with each other. The laughter of children can be infectious. Whatever mistakes Riley and I had made, Shauna and Ryan were beautiful, seemingly happy children. Disneyland *is* a magical place.

Then it was time for them to leave. Riley offered me a chance to go home. But I couldn't. They left. It was harder being without them after that. Depression began to set in, and each day it became a little bit worse. In the shadows of my mind, I could hear the faint calling of the voices who were squirming to get out again. To quiet them, I started drinking. The Richbergs are Orthodox Jews, and they drank sweet kosher wine. I'd sneak a little taste now and then to calm me, and if I had an audition. But now, in an effort to sedate myself, I found myself drinking their wine much too frequently.

One night, while Mrs. Richberg (Gina as she preferred me to call her) was soaking in her massive hot tub, she called for me and asked if I had been drinking her sweet wine. I had to confess. I'd been drinking it to stay normal. I began to tell her about my illness, my relationship with Riley, leaving and missing my children, and how that first episode led to the night at Oakcrest, and ensuing ones after that. I figured she would ask me to pack my bags and leave; instead, she asked to help. I couldn't believe it. I thanked her profusely, and she offered to look at any records I had, evaluate them, and give me her professional opinion.

I had my records in the trunk of my car, where they'd been sitting for months. They made a thick file. I left it on her desk, thinking it might take her a day or two to get through it. But an hour later, she had an answer. "From what I've read in your file,

I would say you suffer from being bipolar." *Bipolar.* Finally, a name. Bipolar. She went on to explain the two "poles" of hyper-energized feelings, mania and its dark and deadening opposite, depression.

Gina was pretty sure, but like any good doctor, she suggested I get a second opinion. I saw another doctor, who agreed and wrote me a prescription for some drugs that would level me out. Knowing that there was a term for it, studies about it, even experts who'd written about it, gave me some relief, but it also made me curious to learn more. With further research, I discovered it is rooted both in nature (my DNA and the dysfunction of my brain) and nurture (what happens in your life, including traumas and chronic stress).

It may sound weird, but now, newly diagnosed, I felt a rush of optimism. My malady had a name, finally something recognizable that could be treated. I worked for people who understood and supported me, and I just knew I was on my way to being cured. All that was left was getting a job as an actress, then a nice place for me and my children. And as far as I was concerned, it was right around the corner. Unexpectedly, when everything seemed so clear, the mania was beginning, and at its peak something would happen to change my life forever.

If you audition enough in Hollywood, you become friends with the casting directors, associates, and basically anyone working for them. I had befriended a young casting intern who got me a chance to audition for an independent film. The director was a dashing Spaniard who was fast becoming the director of the moment. To protect the not so innocent, let's call him Juan. He was as beautiful as Antonio Banderas, but younger and shorter, perfect for my tiny frame. From the moment I met him, I couldn't stop daydreaming about this beautiful man. I asked my casting friend if he was married. She shook her head no. I have to have him, I thought. Then she remembered.

"Wait, he has a fiancée, and they're going to have a baby." That meant hands off, but I still couldn't stop staring at him and wanting him. For the next couple nights, I tossed and turned in my bed, imagining Juan lying next to me. Whether it was just loneliness or lust, I didn't care. I called the casting office to find out if he'd chosen an actress for the part. He hadn't picked anyone yet, she said, but then she made a wonderful sugges-tion: "How about I give you his number, and you can ask him if you're still in the running?" I quickly wrote down the number. My hands shook as I dialed. I was half hoping he wouldn't pick up. He answered on the first ring. "Hello, this is Sylvia Harris. The actress," I said with my most professional voice.

He responded with a thick accent. "Miss Harris. I haven't de-cided yet. But how are you? Are you enjoying this time in Los Angeles?" I was sweating at the sound of his voice, and then, suddenly, without thinking, I confessed to this stranger about how lonely I was in Los Angeles.

"What if we were to go to dinner? Could I give you a tele-phone call later, and we'll make arrangements?" he asked with that thick, heavy accent with which I was falling in love.

My rational self was saying, You should not be seeing an engaged man whose fiancée is about to have a baby, when you have unfinished business in another part of the States and two kids. But my manic self purred, "I'd love to have dinner," into the phone. He later had to cancel—problems with his other movie, he explained sweetly. Of course, I didn't believe him and swore off men again for the rest of my life. But to my surprise he called again.

"There's going to be a cast party for my last movie. Do you want to go with me? You can meet people. That way you don't have to be so lonely." Excited, I tried to play cool. "That would be wonderful."

I hadn't had a real date in years. Not since I first met Riley. I was excited. I reached into my war chest and got as cute as I could get with a short, flirty dress and the strappiest of strappy sandals. I got to the small romantic bistro on Melrose Avenue before him, positioned myself cutely at a table, and waited. Who says I can't act? Juan showed up at 8:00 p.m. sharp, wearing tight black pants and a dark sweater. I kept imagining how dashing a couple we were as we shared a candlelight dinner. He told me all about his life as a director. He had so much to say that it wasn't, to my relief, necessary for me to tell my story. After two hours of flirting, eating, and drinking, which doesn't mix with the lithium I was taking, Juan took me by the hand and escorted me to a little bar down the street for the cast party. Even if I don't get the part, I thought, being his leading lady would be even better. I was in heaven.

The minute we walked into the party, he dropped my hand to become the man of the moment. Women draped themselves all over him, and he made no attempt to stop them. Feeling ignored, I found a seat at the bar alone, ordered a drink, and sat there watching him soak up the attention while I boiled. My mind began to race, and the voices returned. "Somebody put something in your drink. Check out the three chicks at the end of the bar," the voice said.

I looked over at three gorgeous women who had draped themselves all over Juan, my date—no, *my man*. Then I looked at my drink. Of course, they'd poisoned me so they could have him all to themselves. Well, I'll fix them, I reasoned. I'll order another drink.

My head was pounding as I moved away from the bar with my drink to a little table in the middle of the room. Being the great actress that I thought I was, I sat there and began sobbing and crying. And with each emotion, I got louder and louder. People stopped talking to stare at me. The loud din of a packed bar suddenly became library quiet. At first Juan tried to comfort me, but as my frustration grew, he stepped back as if he didn't know me. My heart, as well as my mind, snapped. Even in my state, I could see the scene I was making, but I felt detached from it. I was unable to do anything but watch, as if it were a movie starring me, the overly jealous woman who makes a complete ass of herself in a crowded room. In my head, I begged for an exit.

The voices gave me one. "Run."

I jumped up from the table, dashed out the door, and stumbled onto Melrose Avenue. I staggered down the street, looking for my car. When I found it, I stumbled in, jammed the key into the ignition, jerked it into drive, stomped my foot onto the accelerator, and drove right onto a crowded sidewalk. People, tables, and chairs flew everywhere. I hit the brakes and quickly shifted back to park. Relieved to see that I hadn't hurt anyone, I put my head down on the steering wheel. Suddenly, there were sirens and blinking lights. As I lifted my head, I saw a cop moving slowly toward my door with a pistol in his hand. In an instant, he snatched me out of the car, threw me up against the hood, and handcuffed me. Panting, I told him I needed to get to a hospital.

He and his partner took me to an emergency room where the nurses shot me up with Thorazine, and I passed out. When I woke up, the mania was gone, and they released me. But I'd left a lot of wreckage behind, not the least of which was my relationship with Juan. I wanted a chance to explain what was wrong with me. But first I needed to rest. So I let a few days pass before calling him to apologize. Finally, I got up the nerve.

"I'm a director," he began. "People know me. I have to keep an image. I'm not even from this country. I have to be careful, and I can't be seen with—"

"Someone who is crazy," I said, finishing his sentence.

"We're all a little crazy." He chuckled, then begged off and hung up.

Luckily, being "a little crazy" helped me to avoid serious charges for my sidewalk adventure, but I was certain that my mania had ruined what could have been a wonderful relationship. I never told him about the wreckage I'd left behind on Melrose, and I thought he would never call me again.

And yet, two weeks later, he did.

He invited me to another party. This time, we ended up spending the night together without having sex. We talked throughout the night. I knew I couldn't let myself fall in love with this guy; he was claimed already. I thought, He'll go back to Spain, and I'll never see him again. But we weren't done yet.

"Sylvia, I must see you tonight," said the Spanish accent. "I must." It was a call I wasn't expecting, but I was glad to hear it.

It was another all-nighter at a mansion in the Hollywood Hills. This time Juan tried to be the doting date, getting me a glass of wine or checking on me as he mingled with industry folks. I wasn't having fun. I really just wanted my man all to myself. My unhappiness must have showed.

"Have a few of these, and you'll have a great time," said a woman with a wink, holding a baggie full of magic mushrooms, once Juan stepped away. I had heard so much about " 'shrooms," but I had never tried them. I thought, Why not? A short time later I discovered why not. I heard the same woman that gave me the hallucinogenic yelling, "Hey! Hey! I need some help! This crazy bitch is going nuts." Of course, the "crazy bitch" was me.

I had started to physically accost the woman. I grabbed, pushed, and cursed her. She had turned into an evil spirit. Some guys at the party tried to restrain me, but I got away by running faster than Usain Bolt out the front door and into pouring rain. I ran around with my arms outstretched to the heavens, trying to soak it all in while they were chasing me. But I was too quick for them as I sprinted back into the mansion and headed straight to the dining room. I knew they were after me, and I had to protect myself. That's when I noticed the blue Wedgwood china nestled inside a very expensive, beautiful hutch.

To protect myself from the evil villagers, I grabbed plate after plate, smashing them on the teak hardwood floor. A couple of them tried to stop me, but like a feral cat I leaped onto the dining room table, grabbed a giant bowl of chocolate pudding, then started throwing gigantic handfuls of it onto the creamy white walls. It was as if I were Jackson Pollock (another manic-depressive) throwing paint onto a huge canvas. It was beautiful to me, but frightening to others. Juan finally tackled me and dragged me out of the party, kicking and screaming. He threw me into his BMW and sped down Sunset Boulevard, cursing in Spanish and smoking cigarettes furiously while I watched streetlamps and cars whir by.

"I can never see you again," he managed in broken English, "never." But he still took me to his hotel room, where I passed out. The next morning, as I came down from my mushroom high, we had a screaming match that led to a visit by hotel security. Juan covered for us, explaining that he was a director, and I was an actress rehearsing a role. When he dropped me off at my car without saying a word, I knew we were finished.

It was almost two months later, around Christmas, that he called again.

"I have to see you again. One more time, before I leave America," he begged. "I have the most amazing gift for you." I thought, Why not?

We met at the Travelodge. While he sat there rolling a big fat joint and talking on the phone, taking care of last-minute details before his return to Spain, I sat there watching him and thought, Sylvia, what are you doing? But I knew what I was doing, although I couldn't admit it to myself. I was trying to fill the gap in my life that surpassed even loneliness. I thought this beautiful man would wipe away all the fears I had for myself and sweep me away to some imaginary place in my head. I so wanted him to love me.

"Promise me," I said shakily, "that you will come back to America." He smiled and said, "I just want to spend a beautiful evening with you." His amazing gift to me was him, I realized.

And I accepted the gift gladly. While the strains of Mariah Carey's "I'll Be There" barely escaped the borders of the tiny radio on the nightstand, we made love long into the night. I was his until the next morning, when I woke up to find him dressed and ready to leave America. He politely said, "Thank you," as he closed the door. Feeling ashamed and down, I didn't go home to see my family, my kids, or Riley for the holidays. Instead, I remained in Los Angeles and cared for my AIDS patients.

For weeks, I thought about Juan. My casting friend told me he and his fiancée were the proud parents of a beautiful baby girl. The news sickened me to my stomach. I began to feel nauseous, and thought that on top of everything, I was coming down with the flu. And then I remembered that Juan had summoned me to the Travelodge to give me a special gift that Christmas.

He delivered as promised. I was pregnant. Again.

The pregnancy made me realize I wanted more than anything to be a good mother to my children, but the nature of my illness caused me to make bad decisions. I do not ask forgiveness for this; I accept the responsibility of my behavior. So many people consider a mental illness, especially the kind that seems to come and go like mine, as a weakness of character. I have struggled with feelings of shame and felt like I should be able to control it by myself. But the hazy boundary between what is and what isn't reality makes it difficult for me to even trust myself.

The cruel irony is that the time I am the most confident is when I'm at my worst: in full-blown mania. I am so sure of myself that I don't even begin to question my thoughts or actions.

Sometimes I receive an occasional strand of clarity that manages to filter through an episode and tells me to take my meds, but then I fool myself into thinking that I don't need them because I feel so damn good.

Pregnant and not sure of my mental state, I returned to Santa Rosa. When I arrived home with my news, Riley and my mother shunned me. They were beyond angry and thought I was foolish to have let such a thing happen to me. I was pregnant and broke; my mother rejected me, and Riley, jealous, insulted, and just plain mean, was not going to let me be pregnant with some Spaniard's baby and live with him and our children. Again, even with my "mood swings," an abortion was not an option. I just couldn't bring myself to do it. Somehow, through all of this, my children gave me a sense of purpose and hope. While pregnant, I didn't take any medications for the disorder and yet remained level. In that moment of crisis, my children were my medicine.

With little money and nowhere else to go, I stayed at a woman's homeless shelter for a few nights and then I rented an apartment with some cash I'd managed to save while in Los Angeles. To keep balanced and to get my karma right, I chanted three to five hours a day, and good fortune did follow. I found a great townhouse with a community center and playground nearby for my kids. I went on welfare to pay the bills, and Riley, still furious that I was to have another man's baby, did agree to share custody of our children.

Mioshi was born that September. It was 1993, and our new president, Bill Clinton, was embroiled in a health care debate with Congress. I was busy being the single mother of a new baby with siblings who adored him. Shauna and Ryan were wonderful as Mommy's little helpers, and it looked as if I was getting back to normal. But Riley still harbored hostility. He was very combative.

When Ryan decided to wear dreadlocks like his mommy, Riley objected to it strongly. He hated it. Then when Shauna wanted to color her sandy blond hair to be jet black like mine, he demanded she leave her hair alone. That and other complaints of his made it clear he didn't want his children to act or look too much like me. Whether it was a racial thing or a fear that they might be unbalanced like me, I wasn't sure. As for Mioshi, he didn't exist to Riley. He basically ignored him, even when all the kids were together. And he constantly watched me like a hawk, looking for any signs of mania or depression.

One of the traps of being diagnosed with a mental illness is that people have trouble giving you the benefit of the doubt. My friends and family always assume the worst, constantly asking, "Have you taken your medication?" And then I have to admit if I have or haven't. Either way I often simply say I have, just to be done with it. The proper treatment can level out emotions and allow for rational thought and decisions, but back then I didn't have the appropriate medicine.

During my pregnancies I never seemed to have a problem, but when they were over, it didn't seem to be long before I could feel myself slipping. I'd found a new doctor who loaded me up with Haldol, Ativan, lithium, and Librium. But over the next few years I was still vulnerable to the occasional bout of extreme mania. The pills did nothing to alleviate my uncertainty or the wariness of the people around me.

As things became increasingly tense, Riley and I argued more and more. After one particularly heated session between the two of us, I needed to get away and calm down. I took Mioshi and we disappeared for a few days. We went to The Woods in Guerneville, a popular resort in a tourist area of California. Mioshi was around two years old and I thought it was a good time to introduce him to one of my favorite musical groups, the Grateful Dead. He loved it, the part he managed to stay awake for. I did not tell Riley or my mother, doubting if they would even care.

When I returned and Riley discovered where we had been, he reported me to the office of Child Protective Services. He did it not because he cared about Mioshi, but to mess with me and, as I was to discover, to lay the groundwork for gaining custody of Shauna and Ryan. When the social worker came to my apartment she found nothing wrong, but the stress of it all led to a bad patch of mania.

With Mioshi at my mother's and Shauna and Ryan with Riley, I woke up the next morning as Annie Get Your Gun— the black version. Everyone loves a cowgirl, I thought for no reason. So I put on a pair of chaps I just happened to have, a rodeo shirt, my cowgirl boots, and a hat, then set out for Kitay, a small town in Northern California with quaint little rows of shops, restaurants, and a couple of bars. Not the place where you see any black cowgirls, especially one in the middle of the street, showing off her roping skills, as I swung a belt over my head, pretending it was a large lasso. In a place like New York or maybe Los Angeles, such behavior might barely get a glance. But in the bucolic town of Kitay, it was enough to call the police. I fought with them, and I was hauled off to jail, screaming that I was bipolar. This didn't matter to them. They booked me, and I spent the night in jail. The next day, I checked myself into Oakcrest.

While I was there, Riley, with the support of my mother, who had chosen to take his side in this matter for what she felt was best for the kids, took this opportunity to go to court and seek full custody of Shauna and Ryan. He wanted to go back to Ireland with them, where he said he planned to start a computer graphics art company. I suspected he had been waiting for this opportunity. I didn't know if something had gone sour with his business, but he was ready to go, and wanted to take our kids with him. I was furious, which did nothing to stabilize me.

The custody hearing was a disaster. After Riley testified that I had always been crazy and was a danger to the kids, he proposed to take the children to Ireland, where he and Mother Irene would raise them in a pastoral environment with good schools. I yelled and screamed, not a good idea in court. I told them he was a bad person, and I threatened to blow the whole country up if the judge let Riley take my kids to Ireland. The judge ordered a bailiff to approach me, and I went berserk. It took several people to control me, and I spent yet another night in jail.

Despite my display in court, the judge awarded joint custody with Riley as the primary caregiver. But since the children were to live with him, and he could take them to Ireland if he wanted to, he might as well have been given sole custody. I was awarded visitation rights every weekend. How the hell was I going to visit my kids in Ireland every weekend? And I was the crazy one? I wondered if the people who made the laws for family court were bipolar too.

My mother's position felt like a betrayal, but looking back, I can't blame her. I was a welfare mother with a history of mental problems, which I did nothing to dispel at that hearing. I showed the world that I was an unfit mother. Underneath it all, I knew that I wasn't fit to take care of three small children on my own, and that hurt more than I could, and still can, quite describe. My outburst was as much a cry of loss, shame, and grief as it was a plea for justice. I was sick, and I knew that, but it didn't change the fact that I was a mother about to lose her children. The pain was unbearable.

A few weeks later, in the early fall of 1995, I watched my children board a plane to Ireland with their father. It was a tearful good-bye for us, and when Mioshi asked when he would see his brother and sister again, I lied and said, "Soon, honey, soon." This was one of the lowest points of my life. I had lost two of my children, I was living on welfare, and my mind was in shambles from my illness. I now notice that extreme cycles of mania can very often set in when the seasons change. And as summer moved to fall without my children, I felt I knew what I had to do. I had to die.

I planned it out carefully, and, in typical Sylvia fashion, I was very dramatic about it. I checked Mioshi into foster care, and then went home. In a dresser with three drawers, I placed what I wanted to leave my children, designating a drawer for each child. In Shauna's, I packed her baby shoes (most notably a pair of Chinese slippers flocked with feathers), dolls, my jewelry, and some poems I had written; in Ryan's, his Thomas the Tank Engine toys and books, his cars, and his action figures; and for Mioshi, his stuffed animals. Then I took an X-Acto knife, which I was planning to use to slash my wrist, and dipped it in alcohol. When

I think back, it's almost comical that I felt the need to sterilize the knife. Did it really matter if I got an infection, if I was dead? That let me know on a deeper level I didn't really want to do it.

At the time, though, I felt sure and was about to proceed when there was a knock at my door. Even though my mother and I weren't really speaking after the custody battle, she for some reason, intuition perhaps, decided to come by. When I answered the door she asked: "What are you doing?" I told her I was about to commit suicide. "Oh, no you are not!" she said snatching the knife from me. We talked the rest of the night. She wanted me to go to Oakcrest, but I insisted I was all right. The next day after she left, I found myself on the roof of the building yelling what I don't know. The police came, talked me down, and then took me to the hospital. That's when I called my dad.

It may sound strange that I turned for help to him, the man who in abandoning me years before had triggered the beginning of my nightmare, but I had nowhere else to go. My mother's Crohn's disease was too debilitating to allow her to care for a grandchild, much less deal with my erratic behavior, and I was still furious at her for siding with Riley. Whatever my father's reasons—guilt, concern, or most likely a combination of both—I appreciated him stepping up when I needed him. So I headed cross-country with Mioshi to live with him.

My dad had moved to his hometown of Staunton, a small town of about twenty thousand in the Shenandoah Valley of western Virginia, more rural than urban, nestled between the majestic Blue Ridge and the Allegheny Mountains. There are a number of historic structures in town, and with its quaint shops and quiet streets, it looked to be straight out of a Norman Rockwell painting. With my father's house big enough for Mioshi and me to have two nice rooms, and a solid local school system, it seemed like an idyllic setting for us. However, the harmony of the physical surroundings weren't enough to contain my emotional turbulence.

Coming from the events in California, I was already in a questionable state, and being around my father, even though he was now a recovering alcoholic and had been sober for years, brought up old memories, anxieties, and fears. Before long I found myself yo-yoing between varying levels of mania as if controlled by some outside force. I knew I was shaky and tried to communicate this to my father, but he was unsympathetic. As far as he was concerned, I simply needed to get myself under control, as he felt he had done with his drinking. He couldn't, or wouldn't, recognize that we were two different people dealing with different demons, different diseases. "Just don't think that way" was my father's school of thought. It was hard for most people to accept shifting states of mind with nothing obvious to trigger them. If you were "crazy," you could get over it; either that, or you were too far gone to ever come back. There's not much acceptance of a gray area, where someone like myself swung between stable and unstable moods. Compounding my difficulty was being in a new community with no psychological or medical support.

A few weeks after we arrived in Staunton, I got into some trouble at a local pool hall. It all started when I ordered a drink. "Can't help you," said the beefy white bartender. He refused to serve me. In my emotional state, I didn't need to be drinking, but he didn't know that. I pointed out some drunken people at the bar and asked why they could have a beer and I couldn't. He asked me to leave, and I refused. I had had little experience with racism, but I noticed that I was the only African American in the place. Was it that? Or was I exhibiting some kind of inappropriate behavior that I was unaware of? Or was it both?

When I refused to leave, the bartender grabbed me harshly by the meat of my upper arm. Pulling my hand back quickly, I swung with all my might and punched him in his face, knocking his glasses to the floor. I was lashing out at everything that had gone wrong in my life—my father, Juan, Riley, my mother, and in particular, the faceless disorder that had shredded my life. Of course, the cops were called, and they threatened to take me in for being drunk and disorderly, even though I hadn't had a single drink. I started crying like a baby for my children in Ireland and attempted to explain the whole custody case. Feeling sad, the cop gave me a break. He said if I would leave the bar peacefully and promise not to return, I was free to go. I did so gladly.

I didn't know if I was about to start hallucinating, or if I had already. Caught between lucid moments and the echoes of voices, I feared I was about to slip out of reality and never find my way back again. I was scared, and could only hope I could hold on that night. I needed help. I knew my father wouldn't understand, but I needed to go to a mental hospital. The next day I called the county sheriff's office, and they sent a deputy to pick me up. Leaving Mioshi with my father, I told him I was feeling sick but would be fine in a couple of days. With a few neighbors looking on, the deputy put me in a squad car and took me to Western State Hospital. As the car pulled away, I saw the confusion on my baby's face. He was in Mommy's hell, and I didn't know how to fix it.

Furlong Three

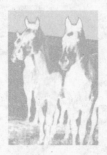

While watching the track ahead, I also glance around to size up my opponents, hoping to detect their strategy. Every jockey is looking for a weakness in his opponent to exploit; is the horse straining or favoring a leg? Does anyone look less than focused? From previous competitions, these riders are familiar with one another. This gives them an advantage over me, but on the other hand I'm a wild card: I doubt any of them know much about Sylvia Harris, so I consider it a wash. What I do know is they don't consider either Pegasus or myself a threat. Why would they? Two losers somehow dropped into this race. What chance do we stand? I consider that my advantage, both for the motivation it gives me and because they will undoubtedly underestimate me. They don't realize I'm racing not just against them but against the insanity that chases me.

Staunton, Virginia

As we pulled up to Western, I began to wonder if I had made a mistake in asking to be taken there. The redbrick building was intimidating in its size and structure. It looked more like a fortress than a place to gain serenity. This was no Oakcrest, which with its modern, officelike atmosphere says you aren't really in a mental facility, but just mentally rehabbing for a few days the California way—low-key, almost leisurely.

This was an old-fashioned state hospital that had been founded more than a hundred years ago as the Western Lunatic Asylum. It was—as the name implies—an institution where patients roam about drugged, looking no less than stark raving mad. As I stepped inside what felt like a prison, I panicked. I resisted the orderlies, who tackled me down onto a gurney. They strapped me in with thick, bandagelike, immovable cotton straps drawn tight against my wrists and ankles. I struggled to get loose and screamed as it became clear I wasn't going to win this fight.

"Give me back my children. Don't let him take them," I ranted.

The sheriff, not knowing what I was talking about, reminded me that my son was with my father. But I kept trying to rip my way through the restraints. Seemingly from nowhere, a nurse appeared with a long, scary needle and injected me with Thorazine. While at Oakcrest, I had been given only one injection to calm down, now I got three shots in each hip. As I drifted off, I clung to the idea that I'd be there for two, maybe three, days tops before returning to my dad's house and my baby, Mioshi. Within minutes I passed out.

I awoke sometime the next day, and although my hips ached like hell, I was feeling level. It was as if nothing had happened; the storm had subsided. Back home at Oakcrest, a stable day or two would be enough to earn your release. But at Western, I discovered, they expected more. First, an initial assessment of the patient is documented, which enables the institution to obtain a court order to hold you until they decide you are ready to leave. You have to show symptom-free behavior for two weeks or more before they will even think about letting you step off the property, and even then it can seem an arbitrary decision.

I had often experienced sadness, regret, even panic, due to my illness, but for the first time since it all began, I was terrified. Was I just as damaged as the patients who roamed the ward, having conversations with themselves, or who were unresponsive, with blank stares, or living in a world only they could see? No, that couldn't be me. The hospital staff didn't agree, and as the weeks rolled by, I wondered if I was ever going to get out.

At Oakcrest, it was about calming the patients. At Western, it was about controlling them. Patients were judged by a point system. Accumulate enough points, and you could get a pass to go home for a day. If you were extra good, you could get more points and hit the jackpot: an overnight stay at home. The point system seemed to reinforce the belief that this was less about an illness and more about a condition you could control yourself; your mental health was your personal responsibility. We were considered more like children who had to be coached into behaving maturely than individuals who were ill and needed understanding. Not only did it look like a prison, it felt that way.

Daily, we went through the same paces. The nurses would

wake us up at dawn. We didn't have to take a shower, but we got points for being clean. Breakfast came next, after which I was assigned to either help clean up the tables or pass out the lists of chores; then we had to line up for our meds. That was mandatory. Later in the morning, there was exercise time, and then an art activity and a quick catch-up with a doctor, who would determine our progress.

The afternoons included group therapy sessions, a smoke break, and then some R & R time to read books in the library or watch the occasional movie in the recreation center, a place populated with people in varying stages of mental decay. At eight in the evening, it was lights out until the next day, when the cycle started over again. There was no room for individuality; being different was what had landed you there. You were rewarded for being a part of the herd, and punished if you challenged it.

I found this out when, after a few weeks, I was sure that I had the necessary points to get a day pass but was flatly told, "No." Mad beyond belief, I gripped a wooden table in front of me, picked it up, then slammed it to the floor. My outburst led to points being taken away, and I was put into solitary overnight for what they called an act of violence. I considered myself lucky. Once, a female patient was caught setting little fires in the bathroom; the orderlies dragged her into a seclusion room where they lined up three straight-backed chairs, sat her on the center one, and tied her to the other two. They left the door open so we could see what happens when you misbehave. She stayed there for three hours, struggling and even soiling herself, before they let her go. To me she was a sick person who was really trying to get help; instead, conformity was more important to the staff. She hadn't conformed, and she paid the price for it. You can get better in an institution, or easily sink into an even more ruinous mental state because you feel so hopeless and afraid.

I ached to see my family, but they didn't visit much. When my father did show up, it was always without Mioshi. I could tell he was uncomfortable seeing me in a mental institution, and I knew he didn't know how to explain it to Mioshi. I was in Ward A. Most of us *inmates* had suffered from similar problems. Age-wise, the group ranged from early twenties on up. There was one lady who, in her fifties, had her first manic episode; she had jumped off a bridge and ended up blinding herself.

I made friends with a few of the other patients. We sat together at lunch and gleefully shared the extra food that was available when someone we knew was absent or just couldn't eat.

There were times we manic-depressives even managed to have some real fun. It is one of the few benefits of the disorder. Mania and delusions can make you feel free and powerful. One time, a few of us put on a show in a little courtyard. We belted out songs for a handful of patients who were the audience. For an afternoon, I was Aretha Franklin, Stevie Nicks, and a handful of other stars. The rush I felt was overwhelming. A high like that is hard to resist.

The highs came less often over the weeks as the staff tweaked my meds. The doctors at Western worked closely with doctors at the University of Virginia, who were testing a syrup made with valproic acid—in pill form it's called Depakote. I had good success with the syrup, especially since it didn't overwhelm me with side effects. Within a month I began to feel good on a consistent basis and was granted a one-day pass to visit Mioshi and my father. The visit went so well that three days later, after three months at Western, I was released.

It was the spring of 1996, and with my new prescription for the "miracle" syrup I was ready, at twenty-nine, to welcome a new life.

I was feeling better than ever thanks to the syrup. No bouts of mania, or depression. Even Mioshi was happier. With my dad around, he had a "father" in his life; someone who cared for him and loved him in his own way. My dad wasn't perfect, but it was better than what Mioshi had experienced with Riley and my mom. I got a job as a waitress at Red Lobster for a few weeks, and then a better job at GNC. For the next couple of months life was good again.

But I was bored. In Los Angeles and even in Santa Rosa, there had always been something to do. But in the sleepy Southern slumber of Staunton, Virginia, there was quiet: acres and acres of deadly quiet. I spent days at home with my father and Mioshi staring out at the pretty countryside, aching for some action of any kind. Even though my father and I were trying as hard as we could to work on our relationship, he still had trouble accepting my mental illness. He didn't understand that the twelve-step program he'd used to pull himself up from the depths of alcoholism is not a prescription for bipolar disorder. But we tried our best, and it helped that I had an aunt and cousins who lived nearby. It was good having family. I hadn't grown up with relatives in Santa Rosa, or with people who looked like me. When I needed company, I walked up the road to hang out with my cousins. We didn't do a whole lot but just enjoyed the hot, hazy days and nights of a Virginia summer, listening to music and eating some good old Southern cooking.

It was during one of those nights that I met Jack. My cousins called him a "white homey," meaning he was a white guy who liked hanging with black people. He was tall and handsome with a warm smile. I liked him instantly. He was fifty, and I decided that was the perfect age for me, someone mature and experienced who probably had tired of playing games. As I checked him out from head to toe and back, a voice, a sane one, said, "It's not a good idea to start a new relationship when you've just gotten out of a mental hospital."

I turned a deaf ear to that voice once Jack asked me to dance. As he pulled me in close, I noticed how good he smelled. His cologne was intoxicating as his strong, muscular arms guided me to nowhere in particular. As we danced, he kissed me. His lips tasted so sweet in that moment. I knew what was about to happen next, and I attempted to warn him so he would stop the nightmare before it started.

"I don't have good relationship karma," I told him.

Jack kissed my forehead tenderly and said, "Karma, like everything else, can change."

"But I completely lose myself in a relationship," I warned.

"Then get lost with me, Sylvia," he said in a quiet voice, and kissed me again.

Cute and corny, I thought. But I couldn't fall for this man. While the music swirled around us, I wanted to tell him the truth about me. But I also knew that telling him I was a manic-depressive could be a deal breaker. While we danced, I danced around my problem.

"Jack, it's been my experience that men are around for a little while, and then they leave." I sighed.

"I'm not like most men," he said, kissing me softly on the lips. I felt safe and wanted.

That was it. I went home with him, and we made love. Jack was a warm and gentle lover. The next morning, he rolled over and said, "I'd like you to move in with me. I know it seems a little insane, but when you meet your soul mate, you just know."

He lived in a small apartment, but he promised to get something bigger for me and Mioshi. We even talked about a future of getting married and having more children. With this man, I imagined a place so secure and serene that nothing from the outside world could ever invade it. He was my protector, my knight in shining armor. I started seeing Jack even more, under my father's suspicious eye. And it was not long after our first night together that Jack bought us a little ranch house deep in the woods of Virginia, on about five acres of land by a pristine freshwater lake.

Jack was going through a divorce. He didn't talk about it much, but I saw that it was difficult for him because he drank heavily. He could polish off a six-pack by himself pretty quickly, but I thought, If this is his only vice and he keeps it under control, then I can live with it. The doctors at Western told me not to drink at all. But I was in love and really wanted to *be* with my new boyfriend, and he hated drinking alone. Together, we drank wine and beer all night and made love passionately well into the next morning.

"I love you so much, Sylvia. I've waited my entire life for you, and I want to be a real daddy to your little boy. He needs a father," he'd say as we cuddled. I was in heaven. I'd finally found what I was looking for: a man to love and protect me, and a father for Mioshi. He even got Mioshi a dog, a little black mutt that followed him everywhere. Suddenly, those horrible days within the gray walls of that mental institution were a distant memory.

I started moving a few things from my father's house to my new home in the woods with Jack. I loved it there. It was so peaceful. As I began to fix up the place, I took my time to make it feel like home, not only for Jack but for me and Mioshi. As with any move-in, the place was disorganized as I went about emptying boxes, arranging and rearranging furniture. But I couldn't seem to get everything together as quickly as Jack wanted. He could still be loving at times, but he was very demanding and old school and militaristic. *Like my father.* And like my father, I found, he could be abusive.

The first time Jack hit me, I sailed across the room and landed on my back. He slapped me hard, and I was stunned. He was frustrated when he came home and I hadn't unpacked the boxes as I had promised. Jack wanted everything put into its proper place right away, and his dinner ready when he got home. All that stuff about being a father to Mioshi ended up to be bull. Jack didn't like having him around and wanted me all to himself. Every night after dinner, he would bark at Mioshi to go to his room, and not to come out until the morning. He never hit Mioshi, but he sure took his frustration out on me.

I had become my mother. It was a turn that I didn't expect.

But I knew how to play the role well. I was a victim, and I suffered as I let this man abuse me. Why? I didn't want to admit that once again I had failed at something. My mental illness had imprisoned me so that I didn't want my family to see me fail at being a mom once again. So I hung in there and tried to make it work.

How I thought I could hide the abuse I was receiving from a recovering abuser was even more mystifying to my dad. In a rare fatherly moment, he suggested that I leave Jack and come back home.

"Somebody here is going to wind up dead, or you're going to wind up at Western for life," he said. He had a point.

By now I was totally without medication and had used up my prescription refills. With the abuse from Jack, I soon became a walking time bomb, and I felt that if I went back to Western for another prescription, they would see my condition and lock me back up. I could feel myself starting to slip away, but once again I thought I could handle it. I wanted to be normal, and as far as I was concerned I was.

And then it happened.

Maybe it was the stress of being with a man who seemed perfect on the surface but was bubbling with anger underneath, or was it that lake? Lakes seem to get me in trouble. I always seem to be near one. It's as if I seek them out, thinking they will calm me. It was at a lake that Riley first saw my illness, and this time it was a tree at the "cabin by the lake" when Jack walked outside and asked, What are you doing? I told him I was talking to an alien. And as is the custom with my aliens, he had warned me of impending doom. He suggested I prepare to protect myself and Mioshi. When the alien comes, he's like a beacon of light that holds me captive as I hear and take in his message. But it was a different picture to Jack. Later that night, he tried to beat whatever demon I saw out of me.

I ran outside and got in my Jeep to get away, but he jumped on the hood of my car, a rock in hand, and smashed the windshield. I got out of the jeep and tried to fight him. It wasn't long before the police showed up. However, they did nothing but talk to us. Once they were gone, Jack broke down and apologized profusely. I should have packed up my stuff and left then, but I stayed with him, hoping to prove my father wrong. I was determined to make my relationship with Jack work as long as he didn't hurt Mioshi.

That changed when one night, in a drunken rage, he beat me to a pulp. Within twenty minutes, my face had swollen to twice its regular size. Frightened, I gathered up Mioshi, jumped into my Jeep, locked it, and slept inside. By morning, he had thrown most of my things into the mud next to my Jeep. I gathered our muddy belongings while Jack watched and laughed. As we pulled away from the cabin onto the two-lane highway, he jumped into his truck and raced up behind Mioshi and me. He tried to run us off the road. For the next ten miles, we raced, swerved, and avoided crashing into each other, all with Mioshi screaming so loudly I couldn't think. I didn't know what to do until I saw a road creep up near us and took a sharp turn. We lost him.

I dried my tears, calmed down Mioshi, and drove him to preschool. Mother and son knew how to put on an act. We walked into his school hand in hand like two people who didn't have a care in the world. No one would have known that Mioshi's mommy's boyfriend had just tried to kill them. A few days later, while Jack was at work, I borrowed my father's pickup truck (everybody in Virginia has one, it seems), went to Jack's cabin, and got the rest of my stuff. I was too embarrassed to move back home again, so I dropped our stuff off at an extended-stay hotel, then went to pick my son up from preschool, hoping to leave Jack behind us forever. But the love story doesn't end here.

He called me at my father's house and at work until I would talk to him. With tears streaming down his face, he told me that he had been a POW in Vietnam and suffered from posttraumatic stress disorder. I felt sorry for him. But I knew that we had a negative codependency thing going on, and I had ignored the signs I'd seen growing up in an abusive home: fighting, drinking, little shoves that turn into angry beatings. It wasn't a good environment for me, and certainly not for my son.

Not too long after that, in 1997, I moved to Washington, D.C., which wasn't too far away from my father and Mioshi. I found work and an apartment pretty quickly. My intent was to get away from Jack and to stabilize so that I could regain custody of Mioshi. My father had become Mioshi's legal guardian while I was in Western. By 1998, I regained custody of my son. I was planning on bringing him to D.C. when Jack showed up. He had found out where I lived and came begging for forgiveness again. He told me that he was broken, just like me. He also wanted us to conquer our demons together.

"Syl, I love you and I don't know why this started coming up in me when we started our new life. We need to try again. I have it under control," he said.

I might be crazy, but the one thing I know I can't do is take care of another crazy person. Jack needed help, and I wasn't equipped to help him.

"You're going to have to go to the hospital. I can't take it anymore. You can't keep beating me to a pulp," I told him over and over again. Finally, with tears streaming down his face, he walked away. But he still stalked me daily, often sitting in front of my apartment building in his car, staring at my window for hours. I just kept ignoring him, hoping he'd go away. Eventually he did, but then something really weird happened. My neighborhood seemed safe until I learned about a highly publicized series of murders that were happening near my apartment. These were grisly cases, with the police reporting body parts like human torsos found underneath some abandoned homes. I wasn't sure if I was manic or just plain scared. Or if it even made a difference.

I lived in fear that one day I would be just a torso underneath some stranger's house. I even wondered if Jack, who was prone to fits of violence, had anything to do with it. It was too much to handle. I had enough money to move, but I had planned to use it to take Mioshi with me to visit Shauna and Ryan in Ireland. I asked my father what to do, and he told me to take the trip. I could come back to Staunton and regroup. I followed his advice and spent two weeks in Ireland. Riley and even his mother were good to us, and, except for Mioshi continually acting out and trying to commandeer all my attention, it was a good trip.

We returned to Staunton and I tried to plan my next move. After having been on my own in D.C., moving back in with my dad proved to be difficult. It was also harder to find work. To make matters worse, in the fall of 1998, while in kindergarten, Mioshi had been diagnosed with attention deficit hyperactive disorder (ADHD). He was put on Ritalin, which only made him act like a little wild man even more. I wanted to take him off of the medication, especially with my own history. I wanted to give him a chance to cope, maybe even outgrow his affliction. But the teacher insisted that we keep him on the medication.

"If you don't keep him on this medication, you're a neglectful mother and we don't want him at this school," the teacher said.

Those words stung me. I'd already lost two of my children, and I was hanging on to Mioshi by a thread. I was not a neglectful mother—at least, not on purpose. I felt helpless to do anything and decided to defer making a decision about the medication until after the end of the school year. Meanwhile, Jack continued to stalk me. He kept calling as many as ten times a day. Sometimes he would just show up on my father's doorstep, banging on the door for hours, begging me to come out. The continual stress of my circumstances triggered my emotions, cycling me into mania.

I had to start another life for me and Mioshi. Whenever I'm manic, I always want to run off and learn something new. It's how I became a nursing assistant, a makeup artist, and an actress. This time I wanted to go to Full Sail College in Orlando, Florida. I saw a brochure and learned it was a school designed to teach different elements of the entertainment industry, from music recording to Internet game design to film production. I wasn't sure what I wanted to pursue, but I believed the curriculum was perfect for me, and it would be a new beginning for Mioshi.

"Are you sure you're making the right decision?" my father asked with concern in his eyes. He knew it was time for us to go, but he didn't want to admit it. He had a personal life too. He had met this woman that he really cared for, and he would never admit it, but we were getting in the way. With me and Mioshi gone, he could get his life back. My father smiled and waved as we pulled off, heading for Florida. But through that smile I saw something in my father's face I hadn't seen in years.

A man who cared.

Furlong Four

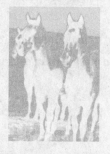

Now the games are beginning. To my right the jockey Miguel is starting to crowd me, forcing me toward Timothy on my left. Timothy knows it and pulls slightly ahead of me to box me in. This encourages Miguel to continue to push me toward the rail. I feel his leg bumping against me, causing Pegasus to edge to the inside.

Most people don't realize how physically punishing racing is. What you see from the stands on your television screen is a graceful picture of movement. But for the jockey, it's a bar brawl. Pushing, crowding, shoving—whatever it takes, you do, and often it can end in disaster. Countless times I have seen jockeys launched from their thousand-pound steeds, then trampled by oncoming racers. Get squeezed against the rail long enough, and your ankle can shatter; if your horse stumbles, you can lose your grip and slide off; if the horse falls on you, it can smash the bones in your leg. When you hit the ground, you may suffer a shoulder separation or even a broken back. There are no pads or protective wear to speak of; your body is on its own. Think about it—most states require you to wear a protective helmet, usually fiberglass or hard plastic, when riding a bicycle. Imagine falling from three times the height, at a speed ten times as fast, wearing only a leather jockey's helmet. Bruises, scratches, and calluses are par for the course. Broken bones and concussions are common; paralysis and death, a distinct possibility.

I am forced to either slow down or go scraping against the rail. Pegasus senses this and slows. I have to regroup before I fall too far behind.

Orlando, Florida

As we rolled into Orlando, Mioshi and I were swept away by this city of lakes. It was 1999, October, right when the leaves were turning and the autumn colors were vivid and inviting, as if to say, "Welcome to a new beginning." Mioshi was excited to be in the land of Disney World, and I was happy to be out of Virginia and away from the craziness I'd left behind. I was determined to be normal. Although we had to check into a shelter, since I had so little money, I knew it would only be temporary, since my brother had promised to send me some money to help me get on my feet.

We checked into a cheap motel not far from the college. One of the things that excited me about Full Sail College, besides the many courses they had in the arts and related industries, was that they promised to work with students in very flexible ways. You could attend part time and slowly build your credits, or you could take advantage of their twenty-four-hour, seven-day-a-week class and lab schedule and get your diploma in the shortest time possible. Years later, I would see that this kind of school might appeal to bipolar students who liked the idea of doing a month's worth of living in a few sleep-deprived days. Likewise, the ambitious plan I set for myself as I left Virginia—find a new home, find a job, care for Mioshi, go to school full time—would be perfect in the mind of a manic individual but at best difficult, if not unrealistic, in the eyes of anyone else. In my overall rush of mania, I hadn't taken the time to think about the details of enrollment. In typical Sylvia fashion, I just showed up at the school without having applied for admission or financial aid. The counselors were patient enough to explain that I had to wait until the next semester. In a way that was good news, because it gave me time to get Mioshi enrolled in school and find us a decent place.

Mioshi, of course, wanted immediately to go to Disney World, which I was more than ready to accommodate. If I had any doubts about coming to Orlando, they vanished when I saw the look on his face as we stood on Main Street gazing at the magical kingdom of Disney. We left that day exhausted as I carried him out, promising that there would be many more return trips.

My brother came through on his promise to send me money, and, after a few more days, I found what I thought was an ideal place to live in Geneva, an Orlando suburb not far from the college. It was a big old house where tenants each got private rooms and shared a common kitchen. It looked out over a lake, and there was a big yard where I imagined Mioshi could play. The neighborhood was safe and pretty, with weeping willows shadowing the street. We shared the house with six women from all walks of life: senior citizens, single girls working in Orlando, and women like me trying to work it all out.

My new roommates and I got to know each other, sharing war stories about bad marriages, children who didn't seem to care anymore, or, as in my case, the difficulties of starting over, again and again and again. During the day, the women all went about their daily routines of working, looking for work, or remembering what it was like to work. But in the evenings we communed at the dinner table and talked about our day while Mioshi pushed around his favorite toy truck or watched his favorite television show. I even made what I thought was a friend there, an older single mother named Susie. She confided to me that she wanted to adopt a child to replace her son, who was about to go into the military. She adored Mioshi and was always giving him little treats like candy or cookies. I felt we were in a good place but, in what had become an ever increasing occurrence in my life, it proved to be of short duration.

New to the area, I didn't know where to find psychiatric help. I was reluctant to ask, not wanting to reveal my condition to others, but also I didn't want to deal with it. I felt I was in control, until I began to cycle toward mania. I tried a community health center program where they gave me meds free, one perk of my low-income status in life, but not the meds I'd gotten from the hospital. The medicine I needed wasn't even in their program; they told me it was too expensive, the drawback to my perk. I took the substitute pills, but they weren't keeping me level, and the manic moments started to begin. My meds were no longer my shield. I did everything I could think of to stop it, but I could feel the mania rising. I tried running, meditating, chanting, reading—anything that would take my mind away from me. But without medication, I was one step away from exploding.

One day I struggled to stay level by cleaning the bathroom, scrubbing it over and over again. Mioshi wanted me to take him outside to the lake. We had been living in the house for about two weeks, and although he liked the other ladies, he was having trouble adjusting to living in a smaller private space with me. It was also hard to share the common areas of the house with strangers, quite different from when we lived with my father in Virginia.

That day Mioshi grew more and more upset and demanding. I told him to wait, and if he helped me finish cleaning, the job would go faster. No five-year-old boy wants to clean a bathroom, and Mioshi, who had a temper, let me know it. He also told me that he didn't like where we were living. He yelled, and I raised my voice in an attempt to control the situation. Screaming matches were not unusual between Mioshi and me, especially if I was manic. But it would pass—we'd hug, kiss, and make up until the next explosion. However, what was normal for us was not for one of my housemates, who showed up banging on my door. I knew there was trouble waiting on the other side of it, but I jerked it open anyway. It was Susie, hands on her hips, trying to peek inside my room.

"What are you doing to him?" she demanded. "Are you hurting him?" I reacted with anger and defensiveness. I told her I had yelled at him, but I certainly didn't abuse him.

"I hate you!" Mioshi screamed from within the room.

"Mioshi?" Susie inquired. The concern in her voice was quite evident.

"Excuse me," I said. "He's five, and he was yelling because he doesn't want to do his chores. Please allow us to deal with our own business." With that, I closed the door on her. Mioshi continued to tell me how much he hated me, then started crying. I was too afraid to say anything else, concerned I would lose it. I went back to cleaning the bathroom, while he cried on the bed.

Later that day, I received more visitors. Annoyed, I swung the door open again. But this time there was a social worker and a male police officer waiting at the other end. Susie had accused me of being drunk and beating my son with a belt. She said that I told him, "Clean this fucking room." I denied it all. I didn't recall speaking to my son in that manner, and I was offended at the accusation. To tell the truth, I was in a full-blown manic phase; anything could have come out of my mouth. But one thing I knew for sure, I didn't hit him with a belt.

"I've never used a belt on my son. I don't own a belt. You can go in my Jeep and check my things. Where did I hit him with a belt? Show me. Check him and show me some evidence of me beating him with a belt." My belligerence did little to help my case, but I couldn't help it. I was angry.

The social worker said she needed to talk to Mioshi alone. The officer, followed by the social worker, took Mioshi downstairs to the kitchen, where he ate milk and cookies while being interrogated. I waited in my room patiently. Minutes felt like days as I waited for the officer and the social worker to return with my child. When they did, I could tell from the look on the social worker's face that it wasn't going to be good.

"Mioshi said you hit him with a belt," the social worker said in a low voice.

"He said I hit him with a belt?" I repeated, bewildered and lost for words. "He's lying," I explained. "He's been doing that a lot lately when he can't get his way." Then the social worker hit me with an even bigger bombshell. She asked whether I had a history of mental illness. I admitted to being bipolar, but promised her I had never harmed my children.

"I don't feel entirely comfortable leaving this child with you, Miss Harris," she said. "He goes to foster care until we can straighten out this mess."

I could see that the social worker felt bad for me, and she was just doing her job. The situation was sticky because I had convinced my dad to let me bring Mioshi on my new adventure. Now, Child Protective Services in two states would be deciding our future. It wasn't looking too bright. When I went downstairs to see Mioshi, he was having fun with his new best friend, the police officer. He glanced at me and smiled in a way that said, "I'm getting back at Mommy for not taking me to the lake." Mioshi was too young to understand the dangerous game he was playing. And even though I didn't want him to go to Child Protective Services, I knew the truth. I was manic without medication. A few days away from Mioshi would give me some time to get it together. I had to find a job and some meds to level me off.

As they took Mioshi away, I wanted to hug him and squeeze him to let him know how much I loved him. But he was happy getting the attention he had been seeking, and he showed it as he walked to the patrol car, putting his thumbs in his ears and sticking out his tongue at me. The landlady ran up to me and handed me back my rent money. She was flustered. "Miss Harris, I want you to go today. You must go. This is far too disruptive."

I was left with no place to stay and no one to turn to. As a mother who had just lost her child, I was overwhelmed with feelings of grief and shame. The manic feelings now started to roar in my mind like a jet engine. I was flooded with a sense of outrage and an urgent, desperate desire to find someplace where I might be understood and treated fairly. I stumbled across a small clinic where they admitted me for a couple of days and administered Thorazine. I felt better, but Thorazine, of course, doesn't change reality. Once I got out of the clinic, I still had to deal with the fact that I was without a home and without my son. Mioshi was in temporary foster care, and the child welfare authorities assured me that if I met certain requirements, we would be reunited. I found a place in Stanford, another Orlando suburb. It was a two-bedroom, partially furnished apartment in a small house broken up into three rental units.

I met the landlady, Myrna. She was Haitian and seemed nice enough. She showed me to the apartment and asked for three months' rent in advance. I gave her what was left of the money returned from the previous landlady and settled in. This may sound funny, coming from me, but Myrna was a little touched. There was something odd about her. She was a single mom like me, with a six-year-old son. We had a lot in common, and yet I felt a need to keep my distance from her, mainly because I didn't want to expose her to my illness. But Myrna seemed like she was on edge too, as if at any minute she would explode. I recognized it and wondered if she could see it in me. Still, I had to get Mioshi back, and having a decent place to live was the first step.

Next was to find a job, which I managed to do as a docent at the Central Florida Zoo. I was to inform, educate, and guide tours, mostly children, at the zoo. With my love for animals, it was the perfect job for me. I would look forward every morning to being around them. Animals are real and honest, and don't judge. They were often my only friends, showing me affection and care when I needed it the most. I was at home in the zoo with animals of all kinds, even though I hated them being caged. I told myself that they were there for us to learn from, and that some good would come from their captivity. And I needed a job.

I started attending parenting classes, and best of all, the investigation into Susie's accusation—that I had abused my son—ended with a finding in my favor. As far as the agency was concerned, Susie's claims were false. But they still considered me a bit of a risk because of my diagnosis, so they treated me with skepticism and prejudice.

During this time Mioshi stayed with a family that had a house full of children. They were good people, but hardly perfect. Once, the mother in the family, who was probably fed up with Mioshi's challenging behavior, growled at him and said, "I'm gonna knock you out if you don't stop it." The way I saw it, if Mioshi's foster mother could be trusted as a parent, then I certainly deserved to be trusted.

After a month, the social worker came by for an inspection and was impressed. She said I was on the right track and agreed to let Mioshi have overnight visits with me. Mioshi and

I started seeing each other right away. But my time with Mioshi was unpredictable. Sometimes we'd have fun, play games, and enjoy being mother and son. Then other visits were filled with his resentment toward me for all that had happened. He'd been through a lot, and I was hoping that we'd move through this little rough patch and get back on the road to normal. But you can't get back to normal when living in a crazy situation. Myrna *was* touched. She proved it to me the day I looked out of my door to find her pacing on the front lawn.

"Sylvia, we need to have a serious talk," she said in a clipped tone.

I stepped outside.

"I know what your son did. He rode my son's bike. We know he did it, so don't try to deny it."

Her son had an electric motorbike, and Mioshi had been admiring it. Earlier, when he was outside playing, he walked up to it and barely touched it. I quickly chastised him for even thinking about using someone else's property and told him to never touch that bike again. While I was talking to Mioshi, I could feel her eyes burning into the back of my neck. We were definitely being watched.

"The bike is in a different spot than where my son always leaves it. Your son is a thief."

"Myrna, that's just not—" I began. She cut me off.

"I think you should move out immediately," she said. "Anyway, my mother is coming in a few weeks. That's going to be her apartment now. And, uh, your son is a thief."

I contained my rage and tried to appeal to her as a mom.

"I need this apartment to keep my son," I begged.

She stood there, glassy-eyed, looking at her nails. Then she sucked in her teeth, turned on her heels, stalked into the house, and called the police. When they showed up, they told me I should vacate the premises per the landlord's request. But they also told Myrna she had to return the rent money I'd already paid her.

"This is a crock," she said as she tossed a wad of cash at me. Of course, she was short.

"That's all I have," she said with a shrug.

I gathered our things once again and took Mioshi to his foster home. I gave him a big hug and watched him run into the house. I found a cheap hotel with a kitchenette and settled in for $175 a week. To get Mioshi back, I had to have separate sleeping areas and a kitchen.

I kept trying to be the best mom I could be. But it kept getting harder, especially when Mioshi started resenting me even more. I was losing him fast, and I tried everything to win his affection. When the zoo put on "Fright Night" for Halloween, I thought for sure he would see me as his cool mom again. The plan was for Mioshi to be brought to the zoo by his foster mother, Amy, and she would let us have our time together, while shadowing nearby.

We walked around the zoo, went to some of the exhibits, and tried to have a good time. I was happy to see my baby boy. But Mioshi was still angry with me. He didn't know why he was mad, but he was mad. There was nothing I could do to make him happy. He fussed and complained as we walked into the spider exhibit. My boss was there, and I introduced her to Mioshi. She asked him if he loved this exhibit. He said no, and then all of a sudden he spat on me and yelled, "I hate you." I explained away his behavior to my boss, and his foster mom ushered him back outside. I followed them out and tried to talk to Mioshi, but he ignored me, clinging to Amy. She apologized for my son's behavior and took him back "home."

That night, I played the day over and over again in my head, which pushed me to a bad spot. I didn't have any meds—not that I felt it would do much good. I knew my boss was going to fire me once she learned I was bipolar, and Mioshi loved his foster mom more than he loved me. My lack of sound judgment, which is typical of people with bipolar disorder, bit me again. Devastated, I quit the zoo the next day, jumped into my Jeep, and headed for Orlando. I didn't see Mioshi again for a long time.

Anyone who lives a stable, middle-class life with supportive friends and family and a secure job would be shocked by the string of disasters I met in Orlando and wonder how it's even possible for so many bad things to happen to one person in such a short time. To understand it, you have to consider all the ways that bipolar disorder can affect a person's life. From that very first breakdown in Santa Rosa, my episodes had frightened or alienated people who might have helped me. At the same time, organizing myself to attend college over a long stretch of time was impossible, which limited my career choices. And my ability to assess other people—the men I dated, landlords, roommates, etcetera—was often compromised. I couldn't seem to detect the signals that would help me avoid untrustworthy people. Finally, many of the decisions I made while under the influence of my mood disorder would haunt me as time passed.

• • •

Before long I ran out of money. All I had was a few dollars and a few clothes in the back of my Jeep.

Without Mioshi, I was considered a single woman. I couldn't turn to the many programs that served mothers with children. And while Orlando offered homeless men several options for temporary shelter, there was nothing available for single adult women. Desperate for rest, I'd drive my Jeep to places on the outskirts of town—undeveloped house lots with thick trees and dirt paths—where I could hide and sleep.

I looked for work every morning at an agency that placed day laborers; sometimes I'd get work, but often I didn't. When I did, I used the money I earned for a room in which to sleep and shower; or for gas, and if lucky, for both. At night, I drank with my new friends who lived in the park. I knew I shouldn't be drinking, but while being with Jack I had gotten used to it. Besides, I wanted to fit in with these people. They were homeless too. Some were bipolar like me, or schizophrenic. Others were alcoholics, drug addicts, or AIDS victims. But when we got together, we didn't judge each other. We were all there because of some rotten circumstances. Some had hope, but most had given up. I was somewhere in between. This is how homelessness happens. One bit of misfortune—bipolar disorder, for example—leads to another and another, until you find it easier to stop trying. I was reaching a point where I didn't care anymore. Manic or depressed, I was always "cute" when I stepped out into the world. But without any money, living in a Jeep avoiding the repo man, getting cute was a fading option. That's when I met Renee.

Tall and pretty, she was a hooker who had been on the streets for years, and she knew how to take care of herself. She wanted to make a deal. She had a room in a house where I could stay when she wasn't using it for "work," and in exchange she wanted to borrow my Jeep whenever she needed it. I thought it was a good deal. It was nice to have a girlfriend. Sometimes we would sit up all night and trade life stories. My life was like a roller coaster, and hers was filled with sex, sometime dangerous johns, and crack. She didn't have a pimp, knew how to pick out her johns, and made enough money to have a home, even if it was just a room.

One night Renee offered me a hit. She filled the glass pipe with white rocks and lit it with a big lighter. She told me to take a long, slow pull. I did as instructed and watched the smoke billow up inside the bowl, then travel up slowly through the neck and into my throat. I felt nothing—maybe because I've taken more powerful drugs to level me off, or maybe being a manic-depressive is more intense than smoking crack. For whatever the reason, I didn't get high in those days; liquor worked better. It quieted the voices. It helped me to forget. It also gave me courage the night I decided to turn a trick.

It was Renee's idea. We were playing dress-up, and she told me I looked good enough to pull some johns. I was hesitant, but why not?—nothing else was working. I found a little outfit in the back of my truck that I used to wear when on the rare occasion I had a date. She helped me put on some makeup, and we headed out for a stroll with the other girls. I felt confident as I switched my little hips from side to side on a street somewhere in seedy Orlando. If I made enough money, I thought, I could rent a room of my own, get a new job, and get Mioshi back.

There I was, hanging around poorly lit streets with other girls in outfits I couldn't stop staring at. I looked pretty good compared to most of them, who were on crack. Hell, I even had all of my own teeth. I was nervous, hoping that my "john" would only ask for minimal service, and then I decided it was best not to think about it. Let it happen. The money would wash away the memory. Cars slowly began to cruise by, and despite the circumstances I felt excited, like a schoolgirl at her first dance. The nervousness began to wane, however, as no one stopped. Not one car horn. Not so much as a "Hey, baby" in passing. I couldn't believe it. What was wrong with these men? I thought. What was wrong with me? Whatever little hope and confidence I had left disappeared that balmy night on the street.

My last bit of self-esteem shredded, I gave up after an hour or so. Angry, I went back to the room to discover my car was gone. I figured Renee had taken the car and would be coming back soon. I sat and waited, then fell asleep, still wearing my hooker getup. The next morning, there was still no Renee and no Jeep. Now I was homeless, without a car, or a job, or any clothes except the ones on my back. I filed a police report, and the officer told me that it might take a while to recoup the Jeep, or it could end up in a chop shop (which it did later). I never saw Renee again.

I was so drained of energy and hope that simply breathing, and putting one foot ahead of the other, was almost more than I could handle. I walked to Orlando's version of skid row, a neighborhood formally called Paramore but known to everyone as Little Beirut. This is where charities operate soup kitchens and churches offer beds for the night. I went there in search of some solid ground where I might at least find some relief from the feeling that I was falling down a hole that had no light, and no bottom.

Every once in a while a shiny rental car filled with out-of-town faces would wander off I-4, lost on the way to the Magic Kingdom, and roll to a stop at a traffic light where I just happened to be waiting to cross. If you were on vacation there in the autumn of 1999, it could have been you, confused about your bearings on Orange Blossom Trail and shocked to find not the usual hotels with fountains and chain restaurants but a tumbledown, dangerous neighborhood. Here, weeds grow up from the cracks in the pavement, and the tropical colors—aqua, pink, coral—are coated with dust and grime. So many street people linger on the sidewalks and in doorways that you can't deny a truth about Orlando that the tourist board would rather hide. People suffer there just as they do everywhere else.

On a good day, I would wake up with the sun in the front seat of a wrecked tractor-trailer, rusting away in a junkyard that had been closed for years. Now that I think about it, the place was probably on Florida's list of toxic waste sites, but at the time I wasn't worried about breathing in chemicals or absorbing poison through my skin. I focused more on the fact that the seat of the cab was relatively clean and soft, like a vinyl-covered sofa. If I got there early enough to claim it, no one bothered me.

The truck could be cold, and raindrops sometimes splashed through the broken windows, but I didn't have any real alternatives. And while I tried sleeping under highway overpasses, it wasn't comfortable at all. First, I had to climb up a steep concrete slope to find a flat spot close to the deck of the overpass. Then, I picked out a spot and tried to rest, but the noise of the road over my head—tires whining, horns honking, motors growling—was just terrifying. Add the choking smell of diesel exhaust and the likelihood of a cop catching sight of me with his flashlight, and you can understand why I preferred to sneak into an abandoned salvage yard and curl up in a truck cab. At least there I could manage to fall asleep, and in my slumber be somewhere else.

Walking and homelessness go hand in hand. While walking, you're in constant search of something: a place to sit, sleep, eat, pee, or chant. Privacy is in short supply when you are homeless, and so is peace of mind. This is especially true in the beginning, when you haven't established a routine or adapted to life in survival mode. When you stand in a line for food, sit on a curb outside a job center, or struggle to relax under the terrifying darkness of the black night sky, your mind starts to rush through thoughts, feelings, and memories. It's something like flipping the pages of a book. You see the faces of the people you have loved and who have loved you. You ache for the loss of these connections. You remember things you did well, and you remember where you failed. You get angry and blame other people. You get angry and blame yourself.

Chanting helped the most. It soothed me, and allowed me to shut out the pain and confusion that had become the menu of my life. I'd found a lake where I would chat with the ducks or watch the cormorants dive for fish, and where I could chant *Nam-myoho-renge-kyo* for hours during the day. At night, I lived under a bridge near a lake, where I would chant again. Somehow I knew that chanting, this ancient form of praise, would somehow save my life. But I needed my meds. I'd been to a county hospital a few times and got some emergency pills, but they were gone, and I didn't have the money or insurance to help me pay for more. I knew no one in Orlando, and I didn't want to be a burden to my family.

At my lowest, a simple act of generosity set me on a new path. Karma is one of the tenets of Buddhism. The popular view of karma can be summed up as, "What goes around comes around." But karma is more than that. It's selflessness. It's the actual act of setting an intention that will lead to a result. One night while I was chanting under the bridge, this young couple walked by. She was sick, gaunt, with sores on her face, standing there in her bare feet. She asked me for some money. I told her I didn't have any. But I wanted to help her.

"You look terrible, are you okay?" I asked.

"Can you just pray that we don't get killed?" she asked in return.

It was as if I was staring at a ghost. She had the shakes. Her companion stared on blankly. I looked down at her dirty, bare feet.

"Do you want my shoes?" I asked. She nodded. It felt like the right thing to do. I took them off and handed them to her. She put them on, smiled, and then they walked away.

The next morning, my head and my heart felt good about my gift of shoes to the barefoot girl. But my feet were cussing me out a blue streak. Soon my socks were wearing down from all the walking from soup kitchen to soup kitchen. I'd become a regular at a few of the soup kitchens in Orlando. As with restaurants, there are good ones with decent food, and then there are bad ones. And just like any hungry foodies, when a new one opens, we all like to try it.

The new soup kitchen stayed opened the latest. When I arrived, I got in line, picked up a tray, and started grabbing food. I ate, and then I lingered. That's what you do when you're homeless and you find temporary shelter. You linger. You sit there and think about your next move. Wondering how long you can just sit here, and where you're going to sleep. I must have looked a sight. My clothes were starting to tatter. There were holes in my dirty socks, and I needed a shower. I'd lost track of time, but I had probably been homeless over two months. As I lingered in this four-star shelter, I noticed a man approaching me. Time to go, I thought.

But instead of nudging me out of the door, he sat down next to me and looked me over head to toe.

"Miss . . ." he said, politely.

"Yes," I answered, politely.

"Aren't you tired of living this way?" he asked.

I couldn't speak. But my eyes answered his question.

Yes, they said. Yes, I'm tired of living this way.

Furlong Five

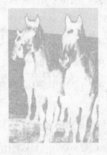

Oraise my left leg and press in deeply against Pegasus's side to prevent it from scraping the railing. Miguel continues to keep me penned in, even though a couple of horses are passing him on the outside. I'm unsure why he seems determined to trap me at the cost of his own race, but I do know there's very little love for me among my fellow jockeys. They feel I don't deserve to be there, that somehow my presence mocks what they do, who they are. But I have no time for that today. I've been trapped enough in my life, and this means much more to me than it does to Miguel. I raise my leg, which is getting ever closer to the rail, and pull it in as much as possible. Then I tap Pegasus to release his power and drive him into Miguel's mount. It's risky, because we may both go down, but I've got to do something. I lean into the neck of Pegasus, who despite the cold is breaking a sweat, and whisper, "What do we have to lose—just everything!" And if I didn't know better, and sometimes I don't, I would swear he laughs.

Ocala, Florida

The minister who ran the soup kitchen suggested I catch the bus that takes the homeless to a place for shelter and opportunity. In my stocking feet, I signed up and hopped on the bus. A group of us stared out of the window as the crowded plastic and neon landscape of Orlando gave way to wide-open country about thirty miles north of the city. The change in landscape from urban to rural was miraculous. Instead of asphalt, concrete, gas stations, and fast-food joints, the land was covered with green grass and dotted with trees dripping in Spanish moss. Houses surrounded by neat little lawns and gardens, small lakes, big swamps, and meandering creeks flashed by. My heart warmed when I saw cattle grazing grass or resting in groups under huge shade trees. It was like going home.

About halfway there, I saw a bald eagle take flight from atop a tower that supported power lines. As it soared through the air so confidently, I felt as if I too were flying away from the life my demons had imprisoned me in. Freedom was near, I thought, as we drew closer to Ocala and I caught a glimpse of horses in pastures and paddocks.

Ocala is Florida horse country. Some of the slow-moving trucks we passed were loaded with baled hay, and in others I could see sleek-looking horses peering through the open windows. Seeing these innocent creatures made me miss my son. I also missed my children in Ireland, Shauna now ten and Ryan, nine. I missed having a life. I prayed that maybe now I could get it all back. There was no doubt in my mind that I was headed to my own Garden of Eden. And I couldn't wait to get there.

The bus pulled up in the driveway of an old white frame house that was worn but painted and in good condition. The small yard in front of it was manicured, and daisies and a few rosebushes grew near the sweeping front porch. A local ministry ran the house and a few others surrounding it for those in desperate need of transitional housing, a fancy way to say "the homeless." It was sort of a halfway house, dubbed "the Ritz" because it was the best one.

In reality, it was a two-story building with bay windows on the first floor and a grand entryway with dual curved stairways. A large antique chandelier hung from an arched ceiling. It had once been a historic hotel, with old state rooms the ministry had turned into small quarters for the homeless. Today, this property has been restored and is quite exclusive, but back then, those rooms had been shut down because they weren't up to fire code. This meant that the eight of us had to sleep in Pastor Al's personal house, which was also on the property. Pastor Al, the head minister in charge, was a friendly fellow who seemed to have had our best interests at heart.

Pastor Al's house was a much smaller structure, and I soon found out that my new bed would be a couch in the living room. It wasn't what they'd led us to believe in Orlando, but it was better than sleeping on the streets. Pastor Al had a strict schedule for his new recruits. Each morning, we were up at six for Bible study. An hour later, we were at a local park for exercise. And we all had house chores. I took kitchen duty and was happy to do it. It was easy to whip up a simple dinner for eight homeless people who had scoured the trash for breakfast, lunch, and dinner. Meat and potatoes or rice was the standard fare.

But it wasn't long before I learned the real reason we were there: we were Pastor Al's labor force for his ministry. The business was telemarketing. And our product was us. We called people and asked them to donate to the ministry so that it could continue to provide services for the homeless. To Pastor Al, we were telemarketers for the Lord, and I was good at it.

"We need to help so many others," Pastor Al, the kindly minister, told me. "Your work here is a blessing for all mankind." I had done this type of work before, and once I got a kindhearted person on the phone and explained that I'd been homeless and the ministry was my salvation, it didn't take a lot of skill to get them to write a check or tuck a few bills into an envelope and send it to Pastor Al's mission.

We worked nine-hour days, which meant that a family would get a call during the dinner hour. We were raking in the cash with our stories of despair. Every day the mailman delivered a huge sack of donations. Sometimes there were so many that the ministry had trouble sorting and depositing the receipts.

Pastor Al encouraged us by promising that we'd be paid a fair share of what we took in. I believed in him and worked hard to persuade good hearts to donate thousands of dollars. I saw the money come in and the checks and cash piled high to the ceiling in the empty bedrooms we couldn't inhabit. Pastor Al promised that the more money we brought in, the higher our personal cut would be when we were paid at the end of each week. I dreamed that my cut would be enough to get an apartment with Mioshi. Finally, at the end of that first week, Pastor

Al gave me my first pay: a crisp twenty-dollar bill. That was it. Twenty damn dollars!

No way, I thought. I'd been on the phone nine hours a day to help get all the money that flowed into this place. From my own calculations, I had brought in about three grand this past week. And now Pastor Al was only giving me twenty dollars? And I was the crazy one? What was I going to do with twenty dollars?

He explained that many of the people they helped were drug addicts, and the ministry didn't want to give out enough cash to tempt them into using. In another time and place, I wouldn't have been able to restrain myself. But after a week of good food, good rest, and otherwise clean living, I felt like some sanity was returning to my life. I could finally see through the haze of just trying to survive and thought, "Sylvia, shut your mouth, accept it, appreciate it, and go find another job." Pastor Al, 1; Sylvia, 0. I let it go, tucked the bill into my nicely laundered blue jeans, and went for a walk.

As I walked through this little horse town, I thought, I can do this. I could make a life here. It was quiet and peaceful. On my stroll, I found the Marion County Public Library. I've always loved libraries, and even in the darkest times I would make a habit of visiting the one nearest me on a regular basis. Libraries are a sanctuary for the homeless. They are warm and filled with fantasy, a place to escape from the harsh realities of the street. One day I went to the newspaper archive and searched Pastor Al's ministry. I found reports on building code violations, unpaid bills, and problems related to his handling of donations.

Apparently I wasn't the only one who had misgivings about this Christian enterprise. Still, I decided not to make a stink of it. While I could condemn Pastor Al, and would have been justified in doing so, something held me back. I think it was the gratitude for the help his organization did offer me and my fellow "telemarketers for Jesus." Of course, he exploited us, and he was probably cheating all those people who answered our calls with donations. But the ministry had also found me in that soup kitchen in Orlando, gave me a bus ride, a sofa, good meals, and a routine that helped me to remember that life offered more than the struggle for mere survival.

Soon after that, the voices returned. They had been threatening for weeks, almost surfacing but then subsiding. I'd been chanting for good karma to keep them at bay, but without any medication, I could only hope for the best. So far my luck had been unusually good, especially given the pressure of being homeless.

I had visitation rights with Mioshi, but Orlando was so far away. I had to spend a few hours on the bus just to be able to spend an hour with him. It was hard to go through all of that travel while trying to get myself mentally and physically back to a normal life, and to do it with little or no money. I needed financial help. I kept calling my family over and over again, but they didn't want to hear from me and refused to answer the phone. Being bipolar wreaks havoc on families; it's like a train wreck every day, hour, minute, followed by a sea of tranquillity . . . a dead calm. But while the manic-depressive rests, the family is left to clean up the wreckage along the way.

Not long after that cry for help, I exploded. My mind raced to the fact that I had been born in Germany, when my mother and father served in the army. I possessed both an American

passport and German birth records. I rooted around my belongings until I found them, and decided they entitled me to leave
America and find safe haven in the land where I was born. In
the mind of an untreated bipolar person, injustices grow to enor-
mous proportions, and the solutions they demand become just as
big. No plan seems unreasonable or unworkable. One morning,
I went to our little local Ocala airport, cut in front of all the
people in line, and practically leaped over the counter, where
this young ticket agent was checking in travelers for flights out
of Ocala. "Take me out of this country," I ranted. From the hor-
rified look on her face, I'm sure she thought I was either some
nutcase or a terrorist who wanted to hijack a plane. "I want to go
back to Germany," I screamed. "I want out! I want out!" That's
what it's like when you are truly manic. You know what you are
doing. It may be extreme, but in your mind it's justified.

She immediately called for security, but the officer was kind
and sensed that something was wrong. As with most manic-
depressives, in time we learn how to cope with our ailment in
our own way. It's like teaching a five-year-old her address or
phone number. You have the presence of mind to say, "I'm lost. I
need help." Instead of saying, "Find my mommy," we say, "Take
me somewhere to get meds." The jails across America, the world
even, are full of people like me who just go over the top, unable
to stop without the help of medication.

"I probably need to get some medication, and I can't get my
prescription because I have no money," I whispered to the officer. I spent that night at a local hospital, which wasn't really a
mental facility, but they knew how to stabilize someone like me
for the night. At the hospital, they gave me new medication, and

even though it wasn't the magic syrup from Virginia, it seemed to calm me down and worked as well. I have to credit the ministry for helping me to pay for the meds.

I was determined not to let this be a setback. I was here in Ocala for a reason; it was my karma. After the airport incident, I continued to explore the town, taking my evening walks around downtown Ocala. One evening during my sojourn, I passed a small storefront with a sign: "Mary Kay Thomas, Equistaff—Now Hiring." When I peered through the window, I saw horse industry magazines on a coffee table. It didn't take much effort for me to realize that this little shop, just a few blocks from the ministry, was an employment agency for all the farms, breeders, trainers, and others who hired people to work with horses.

I didn't know that the horse industry was the most important business in the region's economy, and Ocala was one of the most important centers for breeding and training in the entire world. The area is home to more than nine hundred commercial and private horse farms, and hundreds of other related businesses. While Thoroughbred racehorses predominate, people in Ocala raise everything from miniatures, no bigger than a large dog, to draft horses that can weigh two thousand pounds. More horses and ponies live in Marion County than any other county in America. Only two counties in Kentucky could top the value of the horses sold in Ocala, which exceeds $400 million annually.

All of this requires an army of people—roughly ten thousand—to do everything from mucking stalls to keeping the books. The greatest numbers are needed for the most basic kinds of work, and the demand for these people rises and falls, depending on the season. Many of the horses in Ocala are raised and trained to be sold at seasonal auctions, which means that barns might be full for a few months and then emptied out. Add the high turnover rate of laborers who work with horses, and you begin to understand why farms would need an agency like Equistaff just to keep enough hands around.

Mary Kay Thomas explained all this to me when, after a few days of thinking about it, I finally walked over from the ministry house and asked to see her. Out came a smiling woman who I guessed was about forty years old. Roughly five foot five with brown hair, she was dressed fashionably—makeup, jewelry, dress pants—but without any frills or fluff. She was a no-nonsense businesswoman, and I liked her self-confidence.

"I have a little bit of experience," I told her. Then I described the contact I had had with horses back home when I was a teenager. I was by no means an experienced horsewoman, and I made sure that Mary understood I didn't know much more than how to avoid getting kicked, body-checked, or bitten while delivering feed or shoveling out a stall. "But I love it," I added. "I love just being around them."

"We've got plenty of assignments," said Mary Kay. It was foaling season, and with the population boom, farms needed extra help. She didn't care that I had been homeless and unemployed for several months. The only requirements were a strong body and a willingness to work. On-the-job training would suffice, at least in the short term, she added. But if I thought I needed education in the future, her office provided courses.

The best starting position she could offer was with a wealthy Canadian woman who had brought some hunter/jumper horses to town for two weeks of competition. The employer's name was Angela, and she could pick me up early in the mornings, drive me to work, and bring me back at night. The pay would be about $300 for around fifty hours of work per week. I said yes immediately.

Someone else might dread working with shovels and rakes and buckets, but I thought about the tasks I would perform— cleaning, feeding, grooming—and felt encouraged by the simple dignity of it all. I expected the horses to be as straightforward and honest as all the animals I had known as a child, and the idea of working with them was very calming

I found myself trying to hold back the excitement, worrying that I was only setting myself up to crash. How many times before had I thought I was headed on the right path, only to come to a dead end? Still, something inside me so connected with the thought of horses that it had to be right. It felt too good to deny, so I went with it, despite the underlying anxiety that the rug would be pulled out from me. I even let myself imagine, for just a moment, that I might do well enough to make a stable, independent life for myself, and even get Mioshi out of foster care.

I was pretty excited about my future when I went inside the house and told Pastor Al I wouldn't be available for daytime shifts on the telephone. He seemed genuinely happy for me. After all, the whole point of Christian charity is to help a person to get strong enough to fend for herself. But he quickly added that he expected me to turn over my paycheck to him. It would just about cover the cost of my room and board.

In that brief exchange, Pastor Al revealed his real bottom line. Each of the souls he was trying to save from the streets cost him roughly $300 per week. Of course, even the worst fund-raiser among us could raise that much in a few shifts on the telephone. The rest—many thousands of dollars per week—was tax-free gravy for Pastor Al. Although I had planned to stay cool in my dealings with the ministry, Pastor Al's proposal hit a nerve, and I blurted out something about how he hadn't paid me fairly for telemarketing, and I knew he was facing trouble with creditors and the courts.

"How do you know about that?" he replied in an accusing tone.

Once again, I smartly remembered I still needed the couch and meals I was getting and quickly backed down, acting as if I had just heard some idle gossip. I tried to reassure him that the deal he was offering was acceptable to me, but I didn't promise him that I would just hand over my pay. He relaxed too, and the next morning I was up and ready to go while everyone else was still sleeping.

It was fall in Ocala, and in the pale cold morning light downtown was so deserted you could walk the yellow dotted line running down the center of Silver Springs Boulevard with your eyes closed. I heard Angela's car coming from more than a mile away and was ready when she pulled over to the curb at exactly 5:00 a.m. She waved for me to get in. On the twenty-minute ride to the farm where she boarded her horses, she talked a little bit about the basic chores I'd be required to perform. Though I listened carefully, I also paid attention to the scenery passing by. I was seeing Ocala horse country up close for the first time, and I wanted to soak it all in.

Every road that leads out of Ocala takes you into countryside divided into farms of all different sizes—from a few acres to a thousand—each of them subdivided by fences that create pad-docks and pastures. Some are dotted with live oaks and hard-woods that drip with Spanish moss. Others are decorated with palm trees and sculpted gardens. Occasionally, you'll notice a tumbledown place where just a few horses nibble on the grass in a field and the barns look like they are ready to fall down. But most of the farms are pristinely kept places locked behind big, intimidating gates. Through the trees, you can see barn com-plexes, sheds, houses, and trailers. Once inside the gate, there are big pools where horses exercise in the water, racetracks, and starting gates. And everywhere there are beautiful horses.

Angela's half dozen hunter/jumpers were in rented stalls on a large property where the barns were cleaner than most fam-ily homes. After we passed through the gate and parked near the barn, I got out of the car and breathed in cool air scented with fresh hay and horses. (The barn smell most people find objectionable is found mainly at places where manure and soiled straw are allowed to ferment. Here, and at most places in Ocala, the air was not sour in that way.) Angela introduced me to a trainer named John, who wore a pair of boots that cost as much as a decent used car. I would later learn that John trained horses and riders for Olympic competition. For the moment, he just needed to tell me about the basic jobs I was expected to perform: cleaning, grooming, and feeding.

Most of the time you spend grooming a horse involves going over the entire body with a variety of brushes—coarse to soft—that remove dirt, dust, and bits of hay and also bring out the oils that can make a horse shine. If you are smart, you work from the head down to the tail on one side and then return to the head for the other side so you avoid any possibility of getting kicked. Depending on the conditions, you might also spray lanolin on the horses' coats to keep away flies and other pesky insects.

The trickiest part for a beginning groom involves using a small, sharp hand tool to pick out the hooves. No matter how clean a barn might be, a horse's hoof will inevitably pick up dirt, pebbles, and bits of straw or grass. This stuff gets compacted in the spaces between the hard outside of the hoof, which is called the wall, and a softer, triangular underside part of the foot called the frog. To get an idea of the anatomy you could cup your hand and imagine that the outside is the wall, and the frog would extend from the heel of your hand into the center of your palm.

Horses don't generally offer their feet for just anyone to hold and manipulate. After all, they are flight animals, and their feet are essential to survival. Conditioning a young horse to allow this kind of handling is one of the first things a trainer does, and the horses learn pretty quickly to accept it. Many actually seem to appreciate it, because they are far more comfortable without the compacted dirt and stones that can make it harder to get traction and may even cause injuries and infection. Every trained horse knows that when someone stands close, then pinches a tendon above the back of the foot, that's the signal to lift it. A groom will hold the hoof or rest it on a bended knee, then work quickly to clear out any foreign material. With my little experience, I had seen horses accept this kind of attention, and John reminded me of the steps. But when I approached a massive gelding named Richmond, I wasn't at all certain he would cooperate.

"Rich, this is my first day, so please give me a little bit of cooperation," I begged him.

Then I reached for the tendon on his right foreleg and squeezed it. He shifted his weight to the other three feet and lifted it off the ground for me. I wrapped my right hand under it, and went to work with the pick. As I dug around, bits of dirt fell away, and I could smell the fermented hay, manure. I felt the heat coming off Richmond's body and heard him exhale, almost like he was sighing.

"Richmond, my man," I said with quiet appreciation.

Angela's horses were generally well behaved, which was fortunate for me. Gentle and forgiving, they were patient and didn't seem to mind that I moved a bit slowly as I studied the animals under my care. I tried to get each part of the job done perfectly. Horses are individuals, and while they may share certain behaviors, they also have particular likes, dislikes, needs, and attitudes. Some like to be brushed all over, even with a stiff-bristled scrubber. Others have sensitive skin and would prefer only the softest brush.

I learned a lot from Angela in the coming days and closely watched her train the horses. I also learned barn techniques from this woman, who wanted her charges to be as comfortable and safe as possible. Two weeks later, the job ended, and Angela went back north. Fortunately, my employment agency angel, Mary Kay, had another assignment for me that started right away, and this one even involved grooming horses. The truth was, I didn't have the experience to be a horse groom, but Mary felt I could handle it.

I started at Cardinal Hill Farm the next day, and it was perfect for me. There was a small apartment for me at no additional cost, but I had to share it with another groom, who would arrive sometime later in the season. Still, it sounded like the biggest win of my life. Now I was going to live around horses, and I felt the calmness I'd been seeking my entire life.

A woman named Janice ran Cardinal Hill Farm, and she was a bit more direct than Angela. While Angela was classy with a European style, Janice was a rough and tough horsewoman. From the start, she had a laundry list of complaints. "You're not really cleaning the stalls right," Janice complained constantly for about a week. In fact, my groom's job with her involved no grooming at all but basically cleaning stalls and making sure they were perfect—that and, evidently, listening to her constant sniping.

Maybe she was an unhappy person; there certainly was no love between us. "What am I doing wrong?" I would ask her. "I can fix it." Janice paused for a minute, as if she had to figure it out on the fly. "Uh, you're not cleaning them fast enough," she insisted. She did have quite a few horses, and they were racehorses, which is a whole different scenario than hunter/jumpers. But a stall is a stall, and I cleaned out the muck as quickly as I could before putting down the fresh hay. It wasn't mentally taxing work, but physically exhausting in a way I enjoyed. But there was no pleasing Janice. She fired me later that week for being too slow with my shit-shoveling, to which I replied, "And you're too fast with your bullshitting." I was gone by sundown. Later, I would learn that Janice found two Mexican workers for the price she was paying me. It would be far easier to get rid of me and have two much stronger workers living in her apartment.

Usually, that would've been enough to launch me into one of my moods, but I seemed to be doing better. It helped that I was so focused on getting Mioshi back. Mary Kay took the firing in stride; her own business had been hurt by Mexican workers, who were offering a two-for-one deal across Ocala. I had a little money stashed by then, and thought about getting my own place, but Mary Kay said not to be too hasty. Perhaps she could find me something new before nightfall.

"I have enough money to rent a trailer," I told Mary Kay, who could see how secretly excited I was about finally having a little cash of my own. I had $1,500, which felt like a windfall to somebody like me. But trailer rentals were $500 a month, and if I paid the first and last month's deposit, I'd be back in a situation where I wouldn't have enough money for food or transportation to a new horse job. My angel, Mary Kay, found me another clean-up job at a horse farm, and soon I had enough cash to leave my couch at Pastor Al's house, rent a trailer, eat, and take a bus to work. The next step was to try and get my Mioshi back. I missed him so much it ached, and although I didn't feel it was my fault he was gone, I was ultimately responsible.

I was already dying inside without Shauna and Ryan. I had only seen them twice in a number of years: the time they came to Disney World, and one trip I made to Ireland before I came to Florida. Other than that, it was just an occasional letter or phone call. They were growing up with Riley, and it killed me not seeing my beautiful daughter and quirky middle son. Being a mother is a gift I treasure. Each time when pregnant with my children, I worried about passing my crazy gene on to them, and wondered if I should terminate the pregnancy. But when I see them, I'm reminded that God doesn't make mistakes, even when I'm making them.

I had Mioshi in mind when I fixed up my trailer the best I could. It had one small bed, and I was able to get a sleep sofa from a thrift shop. I covered a card table with a bright blue tablecloth with sunflowers on it and used a large plastic tumbler as a vase to hold the daisies I picked from a nearby field. It wasn't much, but it was the first home I could call my own in a long time. Filled with excitement, one weekend I borrowed Mary Kay's car to bring Mioshi, now eight, out to see what I hoped would soon be his home.

On the ride he was quiet, even though I tried to get him talking. It had been a while since we had seen each other, and we were both nervous. I tried to give him space, although my urge was to hug and kiss him all over. Maybe I should have. Maybe that's what he really wanted, but like delicate flowers, we were both fragile. I wanted everything to be just right.

The closer we got to my trailer, the more I thought about us being together, and how good it would be to have my son back. We pulled up to my new abode. He looked at it and screamed, "I don't want to live in some crappy trailer." I tried to explain that it would only be for a little while, until I could get a nicer place, and at least we could be together.

"I don't care. I don't want to live here," he insisted.

It took all I could do not to cry. After all I had gone through, my son didn't want to be with me. I suspected that the foster mother was turning him against me; I had heard rumors she had inquired about adopting Mioshi. Oh God, I thought. My family isn't going to help me. How can I stop my son from being adopted? I couldn't let her steal my son; he was all that I had left. So the next morning, which was a Sunday, I allowed both of us to just sleep in. I was supposed to have him back by noon, but I didn't make a move in that direction. "Maybe we can go see some horses today? Would that make you happy?" I asked Mioshi, who just shrugged.

Keeping him there was a dumb move on my part; the court doesn't look kindly on mothers who lose custody of their children and then defy the visitation hours. But I was angry; whenever I saw him, nothing was good enough or right enough. I thought, He just needs time with me, his mother, and then everything will be all right. We'll both be happier than we ever have been. Don't I deserve this? Shouldn't he be with his real mother?

By nightfall there was a knock at the door. I hesitated, but knew it wouldn't do any good to pretend that I wasn't home. As Mioshi quietly ate some spaghetti for dinner and watched some cartoons, I opened the door to find, as I had expected, the police.

"Ms. Harris," said an older, disgusted cop, "You're under arrest."

"What's the charge? Seeing my own son?" I yelled.

Mioshi, almost numb to the whole drama, quietly found his backpack and happily went with the policeman. Meanwhile his partner, a skinny, mean-looking man who was almost a kid himself, escorted me to the squad car. I was taken to the station, where I was formally charged with kidnapping. I was released later that night pending a court hearing. Of course, the judge didn't want to hear my reasoning for keeping my son and decided that I couldn't have unsupervised visits anymore; I would have to travel to Orlando to see Mioshi in the presence of a social worker. I was also required to take a court-appointed course in parenting, undergo a psychological evaluation, and accept regular social worker visits for an undetermined period of time. The court did agree to consider taking Mioshi out of foster care and giving him back to me, if I met all my requirements and had a job and a reputable place to live.

It might sound like my actions were the result of another get-wacko episode, but between the meds I was on (when I could get them for free), my chanting, and working with horses, I was doing fairly well. My actions were not driven by my illness; rather they were the actions of a mother desperate for her child. I knew, however, it wouldn't be interpreted that way. Because of my illness, any type of resistant behavior is considered to be the result of my disorder. I am rarely afforded the opportunity to be considered simply human. The benefit of the doubt is nonexistent for a crazy person like me. Yet the fear of losing Mioshi through adoption was very real to me.

I tried not to focus on this possibility; I had to do my job, which was the only way I could stay in the trailer, or maybe save up enough for an apartment for my son. I was sad, but my luck was about to change.

Furlong Six

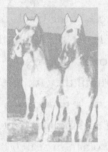

We are accelerating now. My move of coming right at Miguel is working, causing him to turn outward to gain space and prevent our mounts from entangling their legs. As we drive toward him, Miguel takes a swipe at Pegasus with his whip, but Peg is past feeling anything. Once we have driven Miguel to the outside, I urge Pegasus back inside. Free of Miguel and with room to maneuver around Timothy, we power-pass the two of them, speeding after the other mounts and leaving Miguel behind.

Peg's legs are holding up fine. Unlike in our last race, he doesn't seem to be tiring. We definitely have a chance. Of course, I've thought that before.

The OBS
Ocala, Florida

Mary Kay found me work at the Ocala Breeders Sales Company, or OBS, as we called it. At the OBS, they sold babies: horses ranging from young colts to two-year-olds. These horses are trained by older riders until they can get an owner. My new job was not as a rider but as a parking lot attendant, waving cars through and collecting parking fees. Not exactly motivating to a thirty-seven-year-old woman in search of herself while battling a bipolar disorder; so when I could, I'd wander around inside to see the ponies. They were so adorable, but often so rotten. The smaller they are, the meaner they are.

One day I was asked to come inside and help halter-break some of the young colts. I was so excited. Finally, I thought, I get to really work with the horses. But once in, this mean little pony raced at me, pinned me up against the wall, and bared his pearly white teeth at me. I couldn't believe it. After surviving the streets, I was about to be taken out by a little pony. I was terrified.

"Let me out of here!" I yelled to no one in particular.

Dave, the trainer, came over to help me afterward, and I asked him if I'd done something wrong. He said the horse had just been weaned from its mother and was now alone in the stall. In many ways, it reminded me of homeless people in shelters, away from their families. The pony wasn't angry, it was scared, and that was something I understood. From that day forward, I wanted to learn as much about horses as I could.

I asked the trainers to teach me everything. First, they showed me how to put a halter on the ponies—a challenge, to say the least. When you hold a halter in your hand, the pony looks at you with a hooded gaze that says, "Up yours." The best move was a quick whip around, but the ponies could twirl so quickly that suddenly you didn't know if their head or their tail was coming straight at you. Once, a black-and-white baby approached me cautiously and then charged, pinning me up against another wall and knocking the air out of me. I called for Dave, but he wasn't around. Someone else saw my predicament and came running with a broom gripped in his hands. Even while pinned against the wall by this pony, I couldn't take the thought of the baby being struck. I yelled, "What are you going to do with that thing?"

"I'm going to smack it out of the way," said the groomer, who was just trying to be helpful.

"Over my dead body," I yelled.

"That might be any minute now," he chuckled, then proceeded to help me out without the use of props.

I knew from that moment I would never use anything that would hurt the horse. I learned that you can spend thirty minutes with a broom and a whip or one minute with a bucket of grain instead, and they will follow you peacefully. Carrots, apples, and grain work almost every single time with a horse, proving that a little kindness is always better than the whip—a rule I still abide by to this day.

I was a quick study and could see how the ponies would spin to avoid me. But I could still get their halters on without that much push and pull. I knew I couldn't love and rub them, because they weren't having any of it. But we formed a truce of spirits in that little stall, and I came to realize I was doing the same in my own life. Although the job wasn't always what I wanted and I was still without Mioshi, being near the horses had a calming effect on me. I felt I was headed in the right direction.

My duties at OBS varied depending on what needed to be done. I grew to appreciate the grunt work as long as I could end the day looking in on the horses. It didn't matter which one—I loved them all. This was a good time in my life, when everyone liked being around Sylvia, including me. I was fitting in on the backside, the heartbeat of the racetrack.

The backside is where the horses and those who tend to or train them work and live. I was making friends and learning more about how to make a living in the horse world. I used to watch the jockeys with amazement. These miniature giants, some even smaller than me, were great athletes. I admired them but never thought I could be one, until *that* day—the day that changed my life forever.

It was just a normal day in the parking lot at OBS. I was waving my flags around when this older man, small in stature with slim hips and dark brown and gray hair, passed me on a beautiful large brown Thoroughbred. We had nodded hello to each other when he suddenly stopped, turned his horse around, and rode closer to me. For a second, I couldn't imagine what he wanted from me, a mere parking lot worker.

"You know," he said in a low voice while patting his horse on the neck, "I've seen you around with the ponies. You should be up here."

I stared at him.

"You got the right size to be up here—on the horse."

I laughed and shook my head. "Mister, hell no," I said. "I'm too old to get up on a racehorse."

He laughed from his belly. "Well, I didn't start riding until I was thirty-seven. I didn't win my first race until I was forty-two. Let life tell you when enough is enough," he said, then after a nod good-bye rode away.

In Buddhism, that talk was a moment of enlightenment: an awakening, a rebirth. If anyone was looking at me then, they might have thought I was suffering from heat stroke. I was motionless; if two cars had been about to collide near me, I could've done nothing to stop it. I was struck by what had happened. Was it a sign? Was it even real? Had I imagined it? Suddenly it was clear to me: I wanted to ride. For the first time, I allowed myself to actually complete the thought: I want to ride, and I want to be a jockey. For the rest of the day and that night, this stranger's words encouraged me, and I let them run through my mind again and again. *You got the right size to be up here. . . . Why are you too old? . . . Never say never.*

Still, old doubts flooded my mind: Who would teach me? What if I got hurt? Who would take care of me? How would I get my son back if I got hurt on a horse? Who would bother with me? Then my mind focused, and I thought about time, and how I had logged almost a year working with the ponies while working in the parking lot at OBS. I couldn't imagine that the rest of my days could be spent waving a little red flag. My job gave me access to horses of all shapes and sizes, and surely there was someone who could teach me how to really ride on a racetrack as a true jockey.

The next day I started asking around.

I approached a few trainers who looked at me with sympathy, while others just shook their heads as if this was the dumbest idea they'd ever heard.

"You're too old. You'll fall off a horse and kill yourself," said one trainer.

"Ride?" said another, rolling his eyes. "That's a nice dream . . . when you're young. You're so far past the prime of a jockey that the horse wouldn't even let you up on his back."

But one trainer, Rex, was my last stop before I went back to that parking lot and tried to be thankful that I could at least get a job around horses. He was busy working with his horses, but was kind enough to say: "Oh, I know a guy. If you get me a pad of paper, I'll write down the address of his farm. It's around here somewhere."

He gave me the number of an older trainer named Benny, half Swedish and half black. I don't know what difference that made, but he sounded like an interesting guy. Rex said Benny loved to train people of all ages, shapes, and sizes on his horses. For days on end, I kept calling that number, and got nothing. "Horse people tend to move on. I don't know how you could even find him," Rex said. "Sorry, Syl, that was my only hope for you."

Depressed beyond belief, I trudged back to the parking lot. I had been so sure that my eyes had been opened to the true path that was meant for me. Instead, it was only an illusion; maybe it was sunstroke. "Syl, hang on before I have a heart attack." I turned around to see Rex running to catch up with me.

"I ran because I could see how sad you were. You love the

horses, just like I do." He pressed a piece of paper into my hand. "Call Mr. Elmer Heubeck," Rex said. "I know the number's good, and he might help you."

Mr. and Mrs. Heubeck lived on a sprawling horse farm on the outskirts of Ocala. It was the Disney version of my dream horse farm come to life: gorgeous animals wandering around in beautifully landscaped grassy pastures. The property stretched as far as the horizon on each side, and in the rear of the complex of barns and small houses was a regulation-size racetrack for horses. The Heubecks had their own track and backside, filled with horses, grooms, and trainers. I couldn't believe it. My heart pounded as I jauntily walked toward the elderly, white-haired couple while they sat on their front porch.

Mr. Heubeck stood up from his rocker to size me up. "Listen, girl, I don't have anything right now. I'm sorry you came all the way out here for nothing," he said, then folded back onto his rocker.

So much for warm introductions, and before I could say anything, he continued. "I see you don't have anything with you," he said, looking near my feet for equipment. I could barely pay the rent for my trailer, let alone buy equipment for riding horses. "Where is your vest? Where is your helmet?" he demanded. "If you want to ride horses, you'll need those things."

I felt like an idiot. It was bad enough that I had this ridiculous dream, but I wasn't even prepared to make it happen. Fighting back tears, I took a deep gulp of that fresh farm air. Knowing I couldn't afford expensive horse gear, I muttered, "Thank you for your time. I'm sorry to have bothered you," and turned to walk away.

It was over, and the only thing to do was disappear. I continued to walk on the dusty ground, but I wasn't sure where I was going. I headed to the fence line out of his eyesight, where I could have a good cry. Except for the birth of my children, I'd never wanted anything so badly. As I wiped away the tears, I heard him shout something to me.

"Hey, girlie!" Not sure if he was talking to me, I looked around. "Yes, you. Turn around," Mr. Heubeck yelled. "Keep checking back with me." Then he got up from his rocker and opened his screen door, which slammed behind him as he disappeared into his house. I was relieved. I may not have gotten a job, but what I did get was just as good: hope.

"He's a good horseman, and he has an open mind," Rex told me the next day when I explained what had happened with Mr. Heubeck. Rex said to give it time. I did that. But I also did the smartest thing I could do. I started to prepare. I went to a local store and priced a helmet and a vest. The helmet was over two hundred dollars, and the vest was three hundred. Spending five hundred dollars for jockey equipment when I didn't even really know how to ride seemed completely out of the question. I was renting my trailer, and I needed to have a decent place to live to regain custody of Mioshi. Trying to be a responsible mom, I bought a rinky-dink car instead. You could see the pavement through the floorboards. I called it my Flintstone car. It wasn't much, but it was paradise to be able to drive again.

I left my job at OBS and started doing temporary jobs with horses for Mary Kay again. The pay was better, but there was no job security. I supplemented that with home nursing and saved up some money to put a jockey helmet and vest on layaway

Granny and me on my
first birthday

COURTESY OF SYLVIA HARRIS

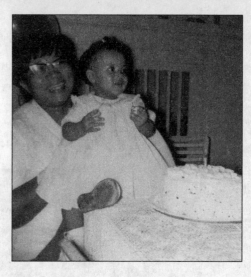

Daddy and the horse that got away with me on it

COURTESY OF SYLVIA HARRIS

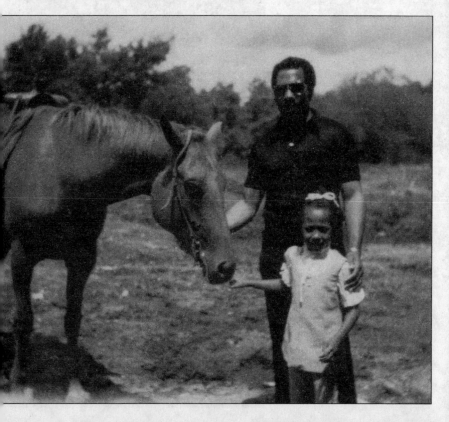

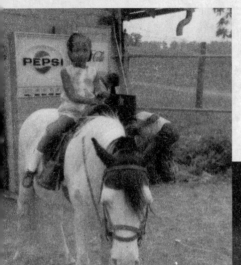

My first pony ride

COURTESY OF SYLVIA HARRIS

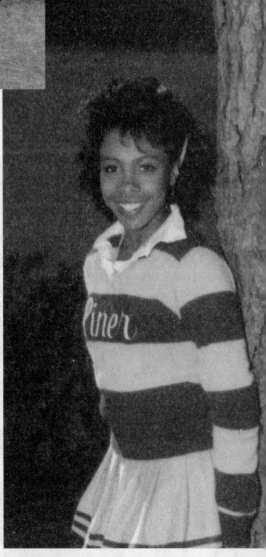

Senior year pep squad

COURTESY OF SYLVIA HARRIS

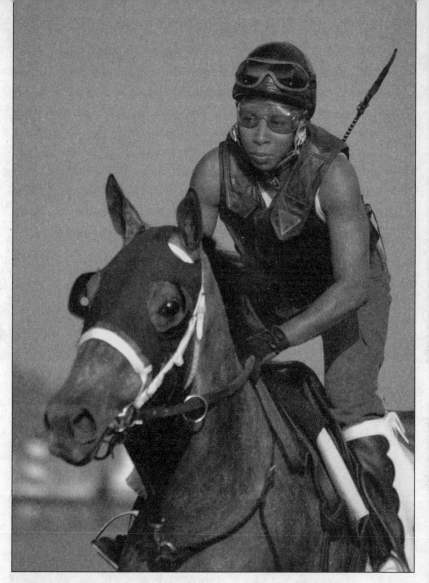

At Illinois's Arlington Park

Nancy Steenhuis Knott

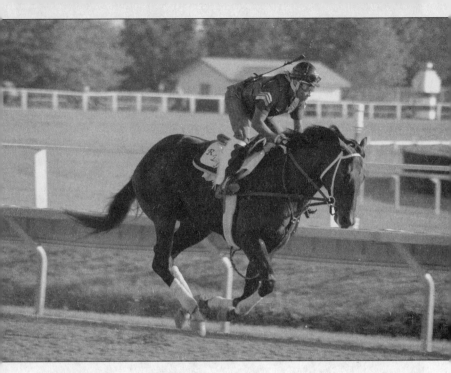

Conditioning a horse at Arlington

Nancy Steenhuis Knott

My first victory

Four Footed Fotos

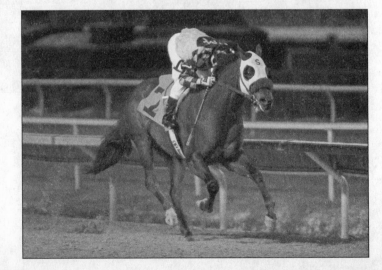

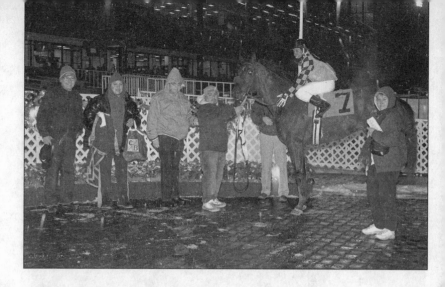

The winner's circle

FOUR FOOTED FOTOS

Win number two

FOUR FOOTED FOTOS

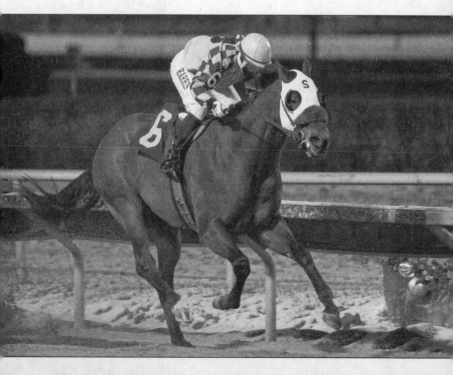

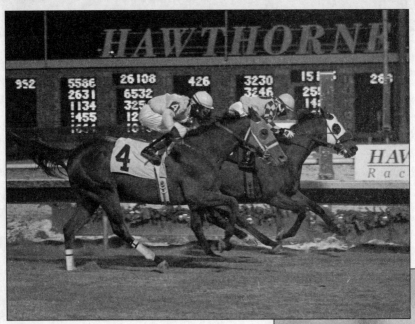

Racing to the finish at Hawthorne

Four Footed Fotos

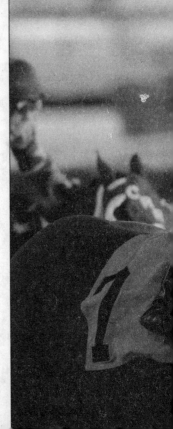

Closing in while riding Rob Why Tee

PETER WYNN THOMPSON

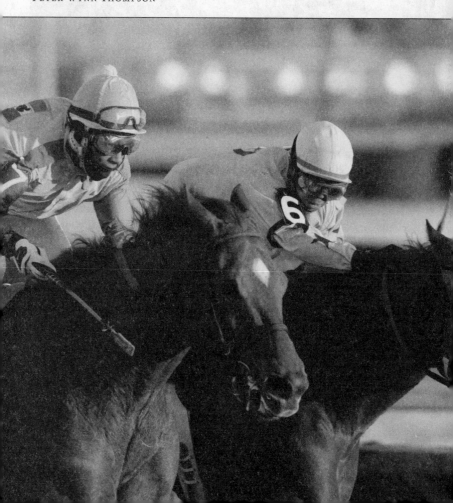

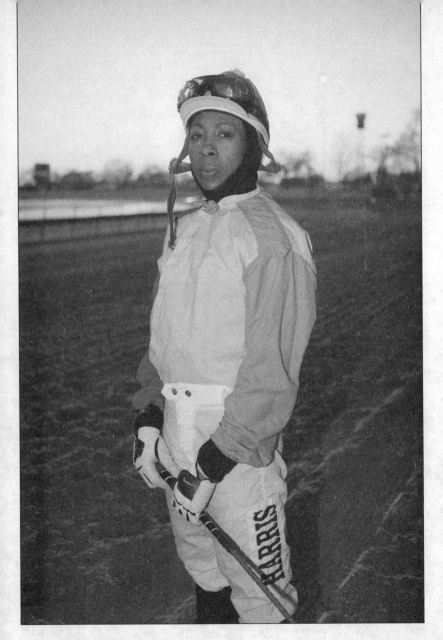

Me, the long shot

PETER WYNN THOMPSON

for $25 a month. It took about six months before I could finally bring my vest and helmet home. I wasn't sure what exactly I would ever do with either. I still had no one to teach me how to ride. But I was also getting excited about having enough money to get an apartment for Mioshi, who was still fussing about living in a "stupid old trailer."

Then another stroke of luck—I was offered a job as a barn manager in Ocala. I couldn't believe it. The job included an apartment over the barn, and even though it was small, it was perfect for me and Mioshi. I had turned the corner, and I thought, My life is finally coming together. I was wrong. One day the farm owner motioned me over.

"Sylvia, you're doing a great job with the horses. I couldn't be happier with you," he said.

"Thank you," I said. "I'm going to learn more and do more. Just give me time."

"One thing," he said. "You do know that we don't allow children here. It's just too dangerous to have kids at the farm. The legal liability is too much for me."

This hurt more than he could possibly know, because my children were on their way to visit from Ireland, and my father and brother were joining us to vacation at both Disney and Sea World. I called Mioshi's foster mother, Amy, and told her that I had already bought the two-hundred-dollar-a-day passes for my kids, and that we were having a family reunion.

It was the summer of 2001. I hadn't seen Shauna and Ryan since Riley brought them stateside to see my ailing mother two years before. That visit had been filled with strife because of Mioshi. The sight of him bothered Riley. He couldn't get over it.

Riley, once sweet and passionate, was mean and bitter. It was as if we'd never been a loving couple.

The court approved the few days in Disney World. On our first day at the park, we waited patiently for Amy to arrive with him. She never did. "I'm sorry," she told the social worker. "I must have mixed up the dates."

I was devastated, and it must have hurt my own father to see his baby girl so distraught. He worked a miracle that day by making a few calls to state authorities. The next day Mioshi, now eight, joined us for an amazing family trip to Sea World, where we jumped in to swim with the dolphins. In a crystal clear man-made cove, my baby Mioshi finally wrapped his arms around my neck and said, "I miss you, Mommy." All the heaviness of my life washed away in those waters. I was with my family, my children, and I was Mommy again.

My Irish twins had grown up so much while in Ireland. They both speak with a light Irish accent, while still embracing their African American roots. Shauna is sweet, with the face of an angel. Ryan is expressive and challenging. He favors Riley but has my fire and wit. There are times when I feel that he misses me and needs me the most, but he'll never admit it. Mioshi, my love child, can be even more of a puzzle. He can be angry, hard to please. We clash, my Mioshi and me. It's as if he's a stalking toreador, egging me on with his red cape, and I'm the bull that keeps charging at him. Of all of my children, he's witnessed crazy Sylvia the most. Being their mother is difficult for me. But I'll never give up on my kids, even if they've given up on me. They know I'm here for them, when I can be.

After a few days of what truly felt like a dream, the time

had come for my family to scatter. My oldest children went back to Riley in Ireland, my father and brother went back to their homes, and Mioshi went back to Amy. Feeling low, I chanted for hours to stem the feelings of depression. I had to make an effort to focus on the progress I had made with Mioshi. Once I got through the pain of the separation, I actually felt pretty good about myself and how far I'd come since sleeping in the cab of an abandoned trailer in Orlando.

As much as I wanted to continue managing that barn, if I couldn't have Mioshi with me, there was no reason to continue. I began to bounce around between jobs and trailers, hoping to find exactly the right setup to get Mioshi back. I had high hopes when I found a really nice trailer to rent in a little town named Citra, not far from Ocala. I had been on the phone at nights, talking to my dad about regaining custody of Mioshi. He had taken a renewed interest in his grandson since the time we all spent in Disney World. I don't know if he missed him, or felt responsible, or just didn't want his grandson in foster care again; whatever, I was glad to have an ally, or so I thought.

It turned out, he wanted custody of Mioshi: He didn't feel I was stable enough to take adequate care of my child, and basically told the social worker and the courts that. Before long I had another custody trial, and the judge declared that it was in the best interests of Mioshi to be with my father. I had done everything the social worker wanted me to do, but my dad painted a picture of me as an unstable mother who would just disappear. I was beyond angry, but what could I say? My history was not encouraging. I knew my father was doing what he thought was best for Mioshi, and maybe for himself, since I think he was missing the little dude. All I could do was watch my father take Mioshi back to Virginia, and try to hold on to the fact that one day he would be back with me. At least he was with family and not in foster care.

I could've gone back to Virginia with them, but I wanted to prove to myself that I could do it: that I could be a jockey or, if not, then a trainer. So I stayed in Ocala to create this dream life for Mioshi and me, and tried to cover all of my bases. The court wanted a more stable job than grooming horses, so I found one selling Craftmatic adjustable beds. It was a sales job that required me to be on the road. But I hauled in $1,500 a week, which was a lot for me. I'd never made that much in a month, let alone a week.

My nights were so quiet and lonely out in the country that I bought a little Jack Russell terrier, Zeke, to be my roomie. Soon after that, I found a new member of the family to adopt. Yes, it would be another mouth to feed, and a rather large one, but I couldn't help myself. One day I was flipping through a horse magazine and saw an ad for a beautiful pony. It was a Medicine Hat pony, also known as a Paint horse. He had dark ears and a mask coming down on his face similar to a hat, and his chest markings looked like a shield. Medicine Hat horses are sacred in Native American culture; only the chiefs could ride them. My great-grandmother was part Blackfoot, and I've always had an attraction to the culture. The woman who owned him lived on a street named Dream Walker Path. It was a sign. I need that horse, I thought. It's a magic horse.

I went to see Medicine Dancer. The picture of the pony was beautiful, but in the flesh he looked like a wreck. He was undernourished, worm-ridden, and dirty, with a matted-down coat, but the animal lover part of my soul considered even an ugly beast like this to be a gift. Appreciate him, I thought.

"I really, really want that pony," I told the woman, and then a lightbulb went off. "Would you take payments?" I asked her.

"Just send me whatever you can," she said.

So I sent her two hundred dollars toward my new pony and boarded Medicine Dancer at a simple but nice farm in Ocala. Within three months, you couldn't even recognize him. He was absolutely beautiful and was considered a "looker." I made sure his diet was healthy and I spent hours grooming and caring for him, but I think it was the love I gave that helped to transform him. Several people even offered to buy him, but I said, "No way am I selling him. He's mine." Those words made me smile.

I had Medicine Dancer, Zeke the dog, my cat Shing-Shing, a home, and a good job. If only I can get Mioshi back, I thought at night as I watched my dog frolic under the stars. I decided that maybe the trailer was the real problem; Mioshi didn't like that kind of living. One day I saw a sign for a lease-purchase option on thirty acres of nice horse land, with a small farmhouse. The man who owned the property was from Romania, and we made a deal quickly. I could rent to own the land and the house.

This was a real working horse farm. There were thirty green acres of rolling hills, a paddock, six stalls, and a tiny red dream house that was perfect for a single mother and her son. The little home was a completely renovated barn made out of stone, with stunning Italian tile on the inside. It wasn't big, only sixteen hundred square feet, but anything more would have been too much. I could see me and Mioshi living on this land forever with the animals I would find to join us.

"I just need twenty-five hundred dollars as a down payment," said Michael the landowner. A strapping fellow who was all business, he listened as I explained that I was owed two thousand dollars in bonuses from my sales job. "If you could just work with me," I said. "I can give you a little bit of money today. This is a place I could raise my son and establish a little horse boarding business."

Michael had his own polo ponies in the stalls, and he played "let's make a deal" with me. "If I leave my polo ponies and you take care of them," he began, "and if you pay me nine hundred dollars a month in rent, I'll apply it toward your down payment."

It didn't take me long to do the math and figure that at nine hundred a month, I would quickly be able to cover his down payment. With only two hundred in my savings, I called my family for a little bit of financial help. "I found this beautiful piece of property that I can afford," I began. "I have a big bonus coming up from work. Can you help me in the short term?"

"I just need five hundred dollars more," I said to my brother, who was making good money but insisted that he didn't have any extra. "Let's pray about it," said my brother, who was on his journey of becoming a preacher. Edward Jr. and I grew up in a quagmire of debilitating illness, manic-depression, and alcohol addiction. He could have walked down any road of destruction. Instead, he chose the ministry. It suits him.

My father said that after the expense of raising my son, he didn't have any extra cash for my pipedreams. I don't blame either of them; I had borrowed money before, and wasn't able to pay it back. Yet this was so important to me. For the first time in Ocala, I knew I'd found a home. I went to my mom, although I knew she didn't have any spare change. Again, I tried my dad, and he refused. To cheer myself up, I asked to say hello to Mioshi, but Dad said, "Um, sorry, he's sleeping right now."

It was three in the afternoon. I thought it was strange, but didn't question it. I had to figure out where to get the money. Fortunately, I was able to get an advance on some of the Craftmatic money owed me. I quickly made arrangements with Michael, and called Dad to share the good news. He was pleased for me, but when I asked to speak to Mioshi again, Dad's mood changed. "He's not here right now," he said, sounding as if he was thinking fast on his feet. "He went to play with the neighbor's little boy."

Something wasn't right, but I couldn't put my finger on it. Every January 1, I'd call my family to wish them a Happy New Year. That day is also a major celebratory holiday for Buddhists. But at 9:00 a.m. on the first day of 2002, Dad said Mioshi couldn't come to the phone because he was busy.

"Where can he be now?" I demanded.

"Oh," said my father in his best fake casual voice. "He's out playing."

I wanted to know what was going on. I was still Mioshi's mother, even if my dad was his legal guardian. My father claimed he had to go and abruptly hung up. I called my brother, who had also moved to Staunton. His response was curious, to say the least.

"Let's just pray together," he said.

In desperation, I called Jack, the ex. "So where are you at, Syl?" he said.

"I'm in Florida, where I've been."

"How come you're not up here? Don't you know Mioshi has been burned? He's got third-degree burns all over his body."

"Don't joke like that!" I screamed.

"Damn, if crazy don't just run in your family."

I slammed down the phone.

That blow hit me hard. With my hand shaking violently, I called Dad. Nobody answered. I called my brother, and nobody answered there either. I called Jack back. "Tell me where my son is at and what's going on."

I had just spent my last bit of money on my dream house and those thirty acres. I didn't even have the money to put enough gas in the car to drive to Virginia, where, as I soon learned, my son had been in the hospital for over two weeks, receiving skin grafts.

Mioshi had always been fascinated with fire. As a toddler, he'd run out of his room with his bed pillow and throw it into the fireplace. Buddhists burn incense at an altar to meditate, and he would take the burning incense off my altar and put it on the carpet. When he was put on Ritalin in Virginia, after his behavior had become a problem in school, his fascination with fire seemed to grow, and he began to torch things with matches. I had hoped he would grow out of it, that it was just a phase, maybe a reaction even to my own erratic behavior.

"Sylvia, we wanted you to know when he was all better," my mom said when I called her for help. "We didn't think you could handle it emotionally, and you've been doing so well. We didn't want you back in one of those places." "Those places" was a polite way of saying "the nut house."

My brother then called and point-blank said, "We didn't tell you for your own good."

I called them every curse word in the book and ended each conversation with: "I hate you with every ounce of me. I never want to speak to you again! Don't ever call me again!" I ranted. "I'm done with you as my family!"

Rage consumed me. I wanted to kill my father. My plan was to get in my car and drive to Virginia and kill him. I'd never had that much hate in my heart except that day in court when I learned that Ryan and Shauna would be moving to Ireland with their father. Pure venom filled every vein.

"We didn't think you were mature enough to handle it," my mother begged during a second round of trying to make sense of what happened. "You know how you get upset."

"I should have been there for Mioshi. I had the money!" I screamed at my mom, sort of reinforcing her statement. "Now the money is tied up in this real estate deal, and I'm stuck unless you give me the money to fly out to Virginia."

"It's best you stay where you are, honey."

I wanted to scream at her some more, but I knew she was probably right. With Mioshi in that condition and me manic and angry, it was sure to end in violence. But I wanted to be with my son. My mother was able to calm me down enough to tell me what happened. As usual, Mioshi had been bored and wanted to play with the flames in the fireplace. "Stop playing with fire in the house," my dad told Mioshi, thinking that would stop him from ever going near the fireplace again. My aunt, who was living with Dad to help out, told Mioshi to go outside and play. "It's a beautiful night. In an hour, we'll do your bath, and then it will be bedtime," she told him.

Mioshi went outside and must have made a beeline to a storage shack in the backyard. It's just a little structure where Dad kept his riding mower, the oil, the gas, and his chain saw. Mioshi found some matches, grabbed them, and walked into the night, trying to find something to set ablaze. The best he could do was a pile of dry leaves in the backyard. The leaves ignited like a little inferno. Mioshi knew he would be in big trouble with his granddaddy and auntie if they saw that he'd defied them with fire again. So he jumped in the middle of the pile and tried to put the fire out by stomping on it with his little body.

By then the fire was too big, and it immediately licked at his jeans and set him ablaze. Mioshi knew to get to a safe area and roll on the ground. But that didn't work, and the dry ground ignited around him, setting the rest of his body on fire. Screaming and crying, he managed to run his still-burning body into the house, where he collapsed. The skin on both of his legs and an ankle had melted into third-degree burns.

Although the injuries healed and the scars are minimal, they are a constant reminder of how for most of my children's lives I haven't been there to protect them. This still hurts me. Back then it made me angry. My son was still under the care and guardianship of Florida when he was burned. I kept thinking how they had taken him from me, allegedly, because I had beaten him. But when that didn't hold water, they declared me too unstable. On my worst days, when I was on six different medications prescribed by a doctor for being "mentally interesting," no physical harm ever came to any of my three children. On days when I was completely manic and didn't know day from night, no harm ever befell my children.

Not even in times when I was intoxicated did anything harmful happen.

I'm not justifying my behavior by any means—it certainly isn't textbook parenting. But still, on my watch, none of my children ever suffered third-degree burns. Mioshi was under foster care in Florida when he was burned. None of those concerned social workers took a moment to call me, his mother, to say he was in the hospital, and for a long time that it was touch-and-go. What if my son had died, and I never saw him again? My parental rights had never been terminated, and I had a right to go to my son in the hospital, whether I could have actually gotten there or not.

"Ms. Harris, we don't know anything about it," the Florida social worker told me. "Mioshi is in the hospital?"

"You didn't know!" I fumed. "You're not doing your job, man! How could you not know, if you were checking? He's been in the hospital for weeks! Hasn't anyone gone to the house to check or provide counseling?"

Deafening silence was her answer.

This was the system for a mother who was disallowed her rights because she was bipolar. If I were a substance abuser, or an alcoholic, I would have been treated with more respect by the government, sent to rehab, and then celebrated for conquering my demons. Instead, the social worker and my family didn't even think about the healing power of maternal love. To them, I was still a pariah.

Somehow, through my turmoil and complete loss of faith in everyone around me, I kept my job selling those beds. I moved into my dream house on that gorgeous property and tried to go on with my life, refusing to answer any phone calls from my mother or my brother. I called my father's house, but only to speak to Mioshi. Faith came first, and on quiet nights, at my own little ranch, I would go outside to sit by a tree and chant. My dog, cat, and the six horses that were boarding in the barn under my care kept my mind occupied, and the voices didn't come during this time. They remained silent.

Then, a few days later, I heard a voice. It was my own. It said: "It's time to ride."

Furlong Seven

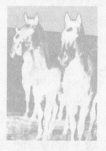

*W*e are moving along at a good clip, but I am worried that the gap between us and the lead horses is too much for Pegasus to make up. I know the feeling. I've been there myself— wondering if I had anything left, questioning whether it was worth it to even go on. But we have each other, Peg and me, and I know that is enough.

At this point in the race, with ground to make up, many jockeys turn to a crop to push their horse to the limit. I couldn't do that to Peg, or any mount. I had my share of whippings in life, and discovered that if you want to get somewhere, you are better off with kindness and support. Without that, at some point, neither one of us would be on the track. We are more than a team; we have nurtured each other and prepared for this moment. Peg is no longer the run-down animal I first met; he is confident, and his heart is strong. I can feel his confidence within me.

"Peg, man, I can't do this without you. What do you say?" Without my doing another thing, he snorts and picks up the pace.

We begin to fly. Love, kindness, and support can cover a lot of ground, very quickly.

Quail Roost II
Ocala, Florida

What happened with Mioshi broke something inside me. I was lost; the pain was numbing. My family kept me abreast of Mioshi's healing, and I was convinced that the best thing to do was to get on the back of a horse and learn how to ride. Yes, a caring mother would have hopped onto the next train, plane, or automobile to rush to the side of her child. I am a caring mother, but I'm not normal. The horses keep me centered. Without them, my life is like a runaway train. I had to focus on learning how to ride. Asking around town for someone to give me riding lessons was futile. Nobody seemed to have the time or the inclination to train me. I couldn't blame them; it's not like I had a lot of money, and who could honestly consider me, a thirty-something black woman, to be professional jockey material?

One day I asked Michael, the owner, if I could ride one of his horses. "My pony is too young to ride," I said, and he nodded in agreement that Dancer needed time to mature. I could ride his horses, but he warned me to be careful. His polo ponies liked to test whoever was on their backs.

Michael chose his top polo pony for my first ride. She was an absolute witch of a horse, and I had no clue. It's true that I had snuck onto a few of his horses at night when no one was looking. Still, I always avoided this one because of her temperament, which bordered on wild.

Michael put me on this polo horse and—*boom*—she took off at full speed. A nasty little mare, she would run straight for things, including going at a dead run toward a utility trailer, veering violently at the last minute to make sure her rider was deposited hard onto the ground. All Michael's horses were high-strung, and when I'd sneak a ride, they would gallop wildly, as if they were saying, "This isn't polo, so there are no rules." The stirrups were a little too long, and this surly mare ran right at a huge oak tree. I rolled off her with ease and didn't get hurt, which was a victory in itself.

"Oh, I forgot to tell you, she can be a little nasty," Michael said, taking obvious glee in the situation. But that was all right. I got back up on that nightmare of a horse. Secretly, I was thrilled because I had taught myself how to roll off a horse, and my body could take it. But this horse was determined to get me. Full speed wasn't so bad, but every time I got back up on her, she took dead aim for a crash job, and I would land on my butt.

It was frightening and exhilarating at the same time. The horse even gave me an admiring glance or two, because she was really trying to dump me. I just went with it. My philosophy is, You don't really need to know what to do with horses. Most of the time, you just need to leave them alone and be in the moment with them.

My dream living situation on this property continued, and except for the worry about Mioshi, my life was complete. I've never been someone who needs or even desires a lot of people around. If I couldn't have that little boy with me, the horses, the cat, and the dog were enough. I was happy rising early to see the sun come up. Watching the sun peek through the clouds always reminded me that it was a new day, and I could hope for peace of mind.

Daily, Zeke would run around like crazy as we checked on the horses, barking, darting in and out, but keeping his distance from any kicks that might silence him for good. He didn't much care to be around the stalls while I was mucking them out. No fun in that, I'm sure he felt. The simple physicality of the chores felt good to me, and with no one there most of the time, I was my own boss. In addition to mucking the stalls, I groomed and fed the horses, making sure they had water and even doing small repairs around the barn.

Walking the horses was my favorite thing to do, because I would engage in conversations with each of them. Who needed people when you could have these magnificent creatures by your side? There was an energy about them that seemed to speak to me directly, with a calming effect. It felt the way I imagined that home should feel. They were my friends, and Medicine Dancer, the broken-down horse I had bought, was my baby. I took extra care of him. Anything I would do for the other horses, I would do twice for my Medicine Dancer. I was determined to nurse him back to full health. The only visitor I had was Michael, who kept coming around more and more. One day he showed up with a truck full of supplies.

"I'm going to build you a round pen for the horses," he said in an excited voice.

I watched him work, and he seemed full of ideas that sunny winter morning. "Sylvia, what if I built another six-stall barn over on the other end of the house?" he said. "I'll have you as my barn manager."

"Barn manager?" I said. "This is supposed to be my place. I'm buying it, so I should be running it." Michael said nothing, and went back to working on the round pen.

When we did the property agreement, I'd trusted him when he said my $900-a-month rent would be applied to a down payment on the land and house. We signed some sort of paper, which I read, but it was complicated and I couldn't afford an attorney to get through the miles of small print. Mostly, I took this man at his word. He seemed eager to get rid of the property and happy to work with me. I was now in the income range where I could afford the property, and my credit wasn't totally screwed. It was just a matter of time and saving until the land was mine, as promised.

I soon discovered that Michael had raised the price of the land without telling me. I still had first claim to the property, but now it was at a price that I would never be able to afford. Michael had pulled a land scam on me, and my high rent wasn't applied toward any down payment. He also avoided paying me wages for taking care of all of his polo horses. I mowed and dragged the field gladly, because I wanted to make the place my home. That was just more free labor for him.

I had been there from January through September of 2002, putting in my money and taking care of his horses. I stopped paying Michael rent, and before long, he gave me a thirty-day eviction notice. Before this, I had made an appointment with a social worker to see if it was a suitable home for Mioshi. I forgot to tell them that I was leaving, and the day after I moved out, I got a call from her.

"I went by your new horse farm, and nobody answered the door," she said pleasantly. "It looked like a nice place," she cooed into the phone. It was. And once again, I would have to tell her that the perfect home for me and my son had evaporated like smoke. It was as if it wasn't meant to be.

I drove away from that property in my brown-and-white Dodge Dakota, which matched my brown-and-white pony: the planned trademark colors at my little ranch. On moving day, all of my stuff fit in the camper of the truck. Earlier, I had moved Medicine Dancer to another boarding facility. With Zeke sitting in the passenger seat, leaning out the window and seeming as sad as I was, I gave the land one last 360-degree look and smelled the gardenias.

I thought about how just a few months earlier, my father had surprised me by inviting me to join him, my mother, and Mioshi at Disney World again. He was extending the olive branch after keeping Mioshi's burns a secret from me. And whether he was extending the branch out of guilt or some other reason, it didn't matter to me. This was a start toward the healing that our family needed—that *I* needed.

It hurt when I saw the burns on Mioshi's legs. But on that day, we had been happy. Mioshi's enthusiasm made me feel like a child myself as we tried to ride every ride and see every show in the few days we had together.

Before my family left, I'd asked them to check out my new ranch. Mioshi was still limping because of his burns, but he tried his best to run around the yard. "Mommy! Mommy!" he yelled. "This is really for us? I can live here?"

Hearing him say that was one of the best days of my life, just as leaving, now, was one of the worst. But still, the image of Mioshi's delight and the excitement he expressed in calling me "Mommy" was what gave me the strength to move on. At least I knew we could share the same dream.

Still, it was tough, and by five the next morning I found myself driving around in the blackness of Ocala with no real place to go. But the miles felt good, and the air zooming through the car seemed to soothe me.

I stopped for a cup of coffee and, atypically, bought the local newspaper. As the sun came up, I started reading the paper to see if there were any rooms or jobs. My eyes went directly to a little ad: "Quail Roost II is looking for exercise riders. Green horses for green riders."

It was the farm of Mr. Heubeck—the same man who told me I needed a vest and a helmet. With the change in my pocket, I called him immediately. Horse people like to get up early, and he answered that 6:00 a.m. call.

"Come out immediately, Sylvia," he said in a warm voice. "I told you to keep checking back with me."

Mr. Elmer Heubeck Jr. was one of the pioneers in the Florida horse racing industry, a giant among those who loved the sport. He had helped build up Hobeau, which was one of the first breeding horse farms in Florida, and now he owned Quail Roost II, a fifteen-hundred-acre horse ranch that included his own one-mile professional track, surrounded by a huge, beautiful lake. He used the track to gallop the horses, and then would often stage his own races. At eighty years old, Mr. Heubeck looked like an old curmudgeon, with his cane and stooped shoulders. Yet this man would end up teaching me what I needed to know for the second part of my life as a jockey.

After lowering himself into his big wooden rocker on his front porch, Mr. Heubeck motioned that I should sit down on the porch swing to talk. There in the early morning, when everything smells fresh, he told me how he didn't board other people's horses and refused to train horses other than his own. Mr. Heubeck had twenty broodmares, their babies, yearlings, and a wide variety of geldings and stallions that lived in his barns and used the training areas.

"I think we might have something for you," Mr. Heubeck said, which marked not only my hiring, but also my blooming. "Do you have the—" he began.

"My helmet and vest are in the car," I promised with a laugh. The minute he told me that he "had something for me," I had as many questions as I had dreams. "Do you think I'll learn how to break babies?"

"We'll get to that, my dear," he said. "I got one or two for you, but I want you to learn how to groom right first."

I started the very morning I read the ad, and Mr. Heubeck spent the better part of the day explaining grooming techniques to me, some of which I knew but many, I discovered, I hadn't been doing as thoroughly as I thought.

"You brush them this way, Sylvia," he said, painstakingly demonstrating each bit of wisdom with his elderly body. Starting on the left side, he used his currycomb or grooming mitt to loosen the dirt in the horse's coat. He would curry in circular sweeps all over the horse's body.

"This is the way you clean their hooves," he said as a large mare nuzzled him and lifted her leg as if she couldn't give it to him fast enough. Mr. Heubeck showed me the proper way to take the hoof pick and pry out any dirt, manure, or anything else lodged in the frog or sole of the foot.

At the end of the day, Mr. Heubeck gave me a smile and said, "Well, the wife has dinner on. See you tomorrow."

And he was gone.

So I got back in my car and slept at the rest stop that night, with Zeke snuggled up against me in the backseat and Shing-Shing at my feet. I had no money and nowhere else to go, but I didn't even care. Despite all that had recently happened to me, I felt blessed and would have lived forever in that car, even on the fringes of Mr. Heubeck's property, if that's what it took to work for this kind-faced man. I went back to work the next morning for another day with my master teacher. The third morning, after finding a nice spot in the field away from his farm to park the car and crack the windows for my animals, I overslept and scrambled to get to work on time.

"Why are you late?" Mr. Heubeck demanded, seemingly more concerned than upset.

My chin sank, my mood went with it, and I decided to tell him the truth. "I'm embarrassed to tell you this, but I've been sleeping in my car," I said in a soft voice. "It's the best I can do these days."

"Oh," he said. "Why didn't you tell me?" Then he took one of his old, arthritic fingers and pointed west. "Go get that big gold key over there for me, will you?"

Relieved, I walked over to the key and brought it back to my boss. He didn't reach for the key, but just stared at me. For a second, I looked deep into his blue eyes and thought about what other horse racing people had said about Mr. Heubeck.

"He's a cracker." "He's a racist." "Watch out for him."

Thank goodness I didn't let that sit in my mind when he said, "Sylvia, I want you to go take that key and open that door over there." He pointed to a door in the back of the training barn. I put the key into a big lock and twisted. When I pushed open the door, I found a small apartment. It was sparse, but clean.

"You can bring your dog and cat," he told me. It touched me that he remembered how I'd told him about my pets the previous day. "I don't need you to pay me anything for the board. But I will ask you each night at eight o'clock to go through the barn, check the horses, and give them their carrots. That's all I'm going to ask you to do. You can also feed the horses in the morning."

It turned out to be a nice little apartment with a shower, a fridge, and a hot plate. He never asked me to pay a dime for rent. Eventually, I would get a few pieces of furniture and make the place one of the warmest homes I've ever had. At night, while I gladly gave the horses their good-night carrots, I thought about how I came to this farm, broken-spirited, only to regain enthusiasm and hope once again thanks to a kindly old man and his elderly wife, Miss Harriet. And, of course, there were the horses.

Once again I noticed the horses had a leveling-out effect on me, similar to the meds I had taken for my bipolar disorder. Being around so many horses and having them fill up my days grounded me. And though I feared another episode, especially because I hadn't had any medicine in a while, I continued to feel good—not the forced high of an uncontrollable manic phase, but rather I felt what I thought was normal.

There were signs of borderline behavior sparked by arguments with other hands on the farm, usually over procedures of some sort. But I felt mine was a natural reaction to what I perceived as jealousy at my treatment by the Heubecks and bias because I was the only woman working with the horses. I thought the other workers were rude, but it never occurred that my own edgy attitude might be somewhat responsible.

One of the most difficult things for me to do is to determine which thoughts and emotions I have are rational and merited by the circumstances. Of course, it's much more difficult to do when not on my meds. Throughout my life I've always thought I could be "cured." And during my time with the Heubecks, I really believed it.

They were like the grandparents of your dreams. Miss Harriet had a little vegetable and flower garden at the back of their house, but she was getting too old to crouch down and dig in the dirt. The first time I saw her do this, I immediately helped by doing the crouching and the digging to plant her flowers and seeds. Miss Harriet was always so warm to me. My first night there, she knocked lightly on my door. I answered timidly. I'd gotten used to bad news and had learned to always expect it.

"You know, dear, I just didn't feel like cooking tonight," she told me as she handed me a carry-out bag. "So I took the mister out for dinner. We brought you back this plate of food. We hope you like hamburgers." I don't know if it was the taste of those patties or the kindness in which it was offered, but those were the best burgers of my entire life.

Each night, I watched Mr. and Mrs. Heubeck walk through the barn and talk to the horses. It was a treat for the horses, and for me too. I would join the Heubecks in feeding the horses their carrots. Mr. Heubeck used to tell me you could never spoil what you loved so much—it just wasn't possible. One day he had a little surprise for me.

"I'm bringing those babies up, and I got one for you to work on," Mr. Heubeck told me.

He might as well have said he was handing me a million dollars. Over the next few weeks, Mr. Heubeck taught me how to start a horse from pony age—that is, introducing it to human touch, bridles, saddles, and so on. I was often invited up to the main house. The home was filled with the fanciest antiques from all over the world, and the warmth of the place enveloped me like a cozy blanket. Between feeding me and making sure everything was fine in my world, Mr. Heubeck would ask me to sit down in his den with his wife and watch the horse races on television. This man, who people said was a racist, and his wife took me in like family, and it was a far more loving environment than the one I grew up in.

I started keeping a little notebook in my pocket and found myself writing down everything Mr. Heubeck would say to me. One night he told me about a special leg paint that I could mix up for horses with injuries. He told me about clays that helped heal injured animals. At first I'd ask him questions, and he really didn't want to tell me any of his age-old secrets. He would finally break down, though, and give me bits of information. And if I didn't push him, he would tell me the rest of it in his own good time, which was how he was with most things.

One day, as I was meditating—I kept up my Buddhism but kept it quiet in fear of what the reaction might be—Mr. Heubeck knocked on my apartment door and asked me to come outside. "Sylvia, I think it's time that you ride," Mr. Heubeck said. I was so excited I couldn't speak.

"You can thank me later." He chuckled.

He took me over to a baby big enough to support a new rider. He was all saddled up and waiting for me. There were no words for the joy in my heart when I put my foot in the stirrup and pulled myself up. Behind me, I heard one of the barn managers say in too loud a morning voice, "She's gonna get that horse hurt; she's gonna get herself hurt." His resistance, I would learn, to a black woman riding would be echoed throughout my drive to become a professional jockey.

"Mr. Heubeck, get her off that horse," said Ned, a big burly man from New Jersey and the head barn manager, who usually got his way with Mr. Heubeck.

"I said she could do it," Mr. Heubeck said in a voice that was final.

With that, I mounted the horse, and he immediately let me know he didn't like it. He swayed and moved from side to side. He wasn't quite bucking, but I wondered if that was next. Mr. Heubeck watched but said nothing, choosing to let me figure it out.

"Mr. Heubeck," reiterated Ned, but a look from the old man shut him right up.

Eventually my horse calmed down, and I got him under control. With my legs grasping him securely, the reins loose in my hand, we headed for the track. I bobbed up and down carefully, growing more comfortable with each stride. It was as if I were coming home from a long trip. Once we reached the track, we began to gallop. When I finished, Mr. Heubeck was all smiles, while Ned walked off sulking. I didn't care. I was learning how to ride like a *real* jockey, and I might as well have been in the Kentucky Derby.

Furlong Eight

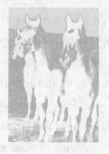

*P*egasus and I take to the outside and turn on the rockets. A
furious blast of snow hits us in the face, but I am warmed by
the feeling of competition.

We bolt past the group of three to the left and then veer toward the rail. The other horses are not about to give up, and
they make the extra effort to gain on us, which they do. Cocky
jocks, all of them male, come up on our flanks; their horses look
Peg in the eye as they gain on us, to make him mad or maybe
just to mess with him like in high school, with the popular kids
always trying to do a head game on those with less. But I'm not
worried.

"Let them think they've caught you, Peg," I whisper, gripping his
mane tighter and continuing our conversation. "No one can catch
you. No one."

Mr. H
Ocala, Florida

My days weren't just in the barn now, but outside on the backs of horses. The ponies assigned to me had spent two years running wild before they were taken to the stalls at Quail Roost II to deal with the most dangerous animal: the human being. While running wild and free in the fields, people sometimes tended to their hooves. But now, much to their initial distrust, they had to deal with me. I'd spend one day with the babies getting the bridle and tack on; another getting them out of the stall; and the next day I'd take them to the track on the property.

In three days, the horse was considered "started." Most riders take a week to start a horse, but for some reason the animals sensed something in me and followed my three-day start plan. Even Mr. Heubeck was amazed that I skipped the usual day or two in a round pen. Horses never go from barn to track and through the gate, but they did for me.

Most of my horses didn't even resist me. Of course, the horses didn't know what the hell they were doing, and in the beginning, neither did I. For the most part, no one really explained it to me; Mr. Heubeck wanted me to find out on my own. I went on pure faith and innocent trust.

There was a big Thoroughbred named Annie who was among the first horses I had to break. I decided we needed to meet, in a mannerly way, in the barn before any of our work would begin. I always talked to the horses; some people don't like it, but I have to talk to them. I place my head close to theirs and speak softly.

"I'm Sylvia, and you're Annie. I really want to help you, so please be a good girl. It's okay. It's not going to hurt. I promise I won't hurt you," I told her that day and every day I worked with her.

"We can do the next part together," I promised Annie. "You just need to trust me." I understood Annie because I had been where she stood—alone, confused, scared, and thinking that someone meant to harm her. The barn manager was clearly exasperated when he would hear me conversing with horses. "For Christ's sake, put the saddle on and just go," Ned would mutter. "Write them a letter later if it makes you happy. We have work to do now."

Ignoring him, I focused on the other three riders working for Mr. Heubeck. They weren't jockeys but rode the horses for exercise to get them race-worthy. Learning from them was one part of my horse education, but listening to my own instincts and to the horse was the bigger part. This was a leap of faith for me. In the past, this wasn't always a good thing, especially when my intuition was often clouded by my disease. But I felt secure with the horses, comfortable, and it seemed to work. The way I looked at it, it was simple. The horse is really my best friend and teacher.

"You break the horse. Let him know you're in control," said an exasperated Ned.

"No, the horse is my teacher," I'd reply. My life revolved around faith, the horses, and Mr. Heubeck.

I was fortunate that the horses accepted me. I'm not sure why they were this open and welcoming to a newcomer. I don't want to call it luck because I think luck disappears, and good fortune remains. Perhaps they felt my own trauma and knew that something inside me had been deeply hurt. Then again, maybe they could simply sense my happiness being around them. Whatever it was, they never backed away from me because my spirit was willing and my kindness was abundant.

To this day, I trust horses more thoroughly than people. You can depend on horses to be truthful and consistent, while my experience with most people has been confrontational, volatile, and unreliable. This would include me too. I certainly have not been a role model throughout my life, especially when manic and angry. But when I'm around the horses, I feel connected to them, and safer than on my own. We're in sync and not at odds, the way life so often feels to me.

After a month or so, Mr. Heubeck said it was time to learn how to gallop. I chose Annie for my initial trial. I put a special yoke around her neck that would keep the saddle from slipping off. Some people call it a chicken strap, but Mr. Heubeck referred to it as a yoke. Riders often hold on to this strap when they ride, but I came to learn that I didn't like this feeling, and it led to one of my more serious injuries on a horse.

It happened on my first day galloping Annie. The day before, jogging Annie around the track had gone without incident, but now it was time to feel her speed and gallop. I had never galloped on a horse before, except for those crazy polo ponies. I didn't know that you're not supposed to stand the entire time the horse is literally flying around the track. But I was so eager to get going that I stood up immediately. It threw off Annie's balance, and before I knew it, I was twisted around with my hand still under the yoke. I had been told to put one finger around the yoke, but that wasn't a good way for me to hold a tight leather belt, so I used my entire hand. When Annie twisted around, my hand—stuck between the horse's coat and the leather—snapped into two pieces. Annie twisted again, and I fell to the ground.

At first, I didn't even know I had broken my hand, because more was busted than just my bones. She busted the yoke off her and got loose from me. Running after my horse with my broken hand folded into my side, I grabbed her, bit back the pain, and managed to get back on and gallop a few laps around the track. I just couldn't let Mr. Heubeck see that something was wrong.

"Coming along, Sylvia," he said. "You're coming along."

The next morning, my hand was swollen to three times its original size, and the pain ran throbbing up my arm and into my shoulder in giant waves. Annie seemed understanding when I got on her that morning and gingerly put the reins in my swollen hand, with the good hand leading the way.

"Look," said Ned to Mr. Heubeck. "I told you Sylvia would hurt herself, and she took a hard fall yesterday. I think there's something wrong with that hand she's trying to hide."

Mr. Heubeck was instantly concerned. "Sylvia, I don't want you to get hurt," he said with gravity. "I think we better wait on you learning how to ride. Maybe we've moved too fast. And I don't want to get sued."

It turned out Mr. Heubeck was a very wealthy man, and he had to be careful. Even though he was a nice, sweet man, he was also the owner of a farm, and lawsuits were commonplace around the horses. Before I worked for him, I heard about what some riders call "the trick" in Florida. When it comes close to summer, a lot of the riders would get hurt on purpose and then file for workman's comp. Some of the more unscrupulous would even sue. Either way, you don't have to work, *and* you have a check coming in. Mr. Heubeck was afraid I'd fall off one of his horses and get myself a lawyer.

There was no discussion, and I stopped riding. More specifically, I stopped riding Mr. Heubeck's horses. When he hired me, Mr. Heubeck agreed to let me bring Medicine Dancer to the farm for free boarding. There, I was able to give him the care and love he needed. Although he'd never be a true racehorse, Medicine Dancer was a far cry from the sickly horse I had bought. I knew he was capable of riding. Forget all of them, I thought. I'll wait until everybody is asleep, and then I'll go ride him. And I'm going to learn how to ride on my own, in my own way, and on my own horse.

Late at night, I'd sneak into the tack room, bring Dancer into the barn, put on his saddle, and ride him out of the barn in the pitch-black with the reins in my now-wrapped broken hand. The pain in my hand was immeasurable, but the joy in my heart masked any discomfort.

For many nights, I snuck into that barn and quietly rode my own horse to the racetrack, but I didn't dare turn on the track lights because the entire farm would have seen us. In the blackness that was our canvas and with just a few stars as our lights, I taught myself how to gallop on Medicine Dancer.

Each night we flew around the track as if ground and heaven didn't matter because we lived somewhere in between. When I was flying, which was what riding had become for me, I didn't dwell on my hand. It had swollen so much that I didn't have knuckles anymore. It was just a padded, distorted something at the end of my wrist. I started taking horse aspirin to knock down the pain. It didn't matter, because I wouldn't miss even one secret rendezvous with Medicine Dancer.

I never again held my horse by the yoke or put that device on any of the horses I would ride in the future. I would just simply lean forward and hold my partner by the mane. The first time I did it, Dancer paused, snorted, and then took flight under that blanket of night stars.

After two weeks of secret riding and pain, my stomach began to burn from the horse aspirin, and one of my fingers bent forward as if it had no feeling in it. Finally, I went to the emergency room, and gasped when they showed me the X-ray of my mangled hand.

"When did you do this to yourself?" the doctor asked me.

"Um, a few days ago," I lied.

"No, you did this a while ago, because it's starting to heal," he said. "You might need to get it broken again and reset your one knuckle, which is healing in the wrong place."

"Oh, Doctor, please, can't we just do something right now?" I begged. So he put a cast on me, but that didn't stop me from riding my horse each night. My horse taught me how to ride, albeit not under the best of circumstances. For the next few months we lived this secret life, and during that time I became a better rider. Once my cast was cut off, Mr. Heubeck, who I suspected knew about my midnight rides, out of the blue suggested I try another one of his older horses. "Just ride it around the barn," he offered, which wasn't the same as asking me to go to the track.

A few days later, he said, "Sylvia, I have another horse back there named Wildfire. You can ride him to the track and do a few laps." Wildfire was a beautiful chestnut, thin and sinewy, and he had promise as a racer. This time Mr. Heubeck watched me ride and offered his expertise. It wasn't always easy to listen to.

Mr. Heubeck was harsh, strict, and cantankerous when he evaluated my horsemanship. "Why are you jerking on that horse?" he'd grumble. "I thought I told you to put that horse over there, and you're over here."

I hated when he was mad at me, and he always sounded angry when he would toss out a correction. He was a man of few words. I prayed for him to say nothing, because that was his version of saying I was doing a fine job. If he shut up, you had it made. That was what I worked for—his silence.

I became like a junkie who couldn't wait for the next horse fix. I didn't care what I got on; I just wanted to ride every single day. Nights still belonged to Medicine Dancer and the moon that guided us. We both grew stronger and healthier. We were each a gift to the other, both of us having been labeled crazy at times in our life. Medicine Dancer had what's called a walleye, which is when a horse has one eye that looks like a white human eye. "Why did you buy this horse with the walleye?" mocked a barn hand. "Don't you know that horses with those eyes are crazy?"

"I like crazy," I told him. "I understand it." We healed each other, and that enabled us to live.

One day, a few weeks later, a couple came to the farm to look at the horses. They saw Dancer running around in one of the pens and asked Mr. Heubeck, "Is this horse for sale?"

"He belongs to my girl Sylvia," he told them, pointing to me.

"I'm sorry, but no. He's not for sale," I said.

"He's just so beautiful," said the man. "I'd love to buy him."

"Absolutely not," I repeated. "Never, ever, ever. I wanted a horse my whole life, and he's my first one. There is no way in the world I'm ever selling that horse. We'll be together until one of us leaves this life."

A week later, the couple came back to see the horses again.

"Are you sure you don't want to sell us that horse?" asked the man.

"Not for money," I said, figuring I'd take Dancer with me and become an assistant trainer while still holding on to the dream of being a jockey. I also wanted to get Mioshi back, and being an assistant trainer for a while might seem like more steady employment to a social worker.

"Well, I heard you might want to be a trainer," said the man. "And in Florida, you can get your trainer's license if you have your own horse to train."

"What does that mean? I have a horse," I said.

The man had a plan. "Why don't you come out to our farm, and maybe we could swap something?" he said. "You can have a Thoroughbred, and I could have Medicine Dancer." He looked longingly at my horse and said, "He has a good head on him, and he's a beautiful pony."

I don't know what possessed me, but I agreed to trade Dancer for a Thoroughbred. Even in the minutes after I did it, my mind screamed, "Sometimes, Sylvia, you just do the wrong damn thing." The Thoroughbred that was now mine was an ugly thing with crust coming out of his eyes, goop in his ears, and he was skinny and small. At first glance, I thought, Hell, no.

Then I thought, "Dancer has been loved. This horse needs somebody to love him."

The wife's name was Debby, and she had been a jockey. I said, "Let's check it out and see if I get along with the Thoroughbred."

She agreed, and I moved Dancer over to her farm and spent time with her horse before agreeing to swap. I still did my work at Mr. Heubeck's, but in the late afternoons I'd go to this other farm to see my new Thoroughbred, Smooky, a horse that stayed put with Debby. I'd mount Smooky each day, letting him teach me how to ride and how to train. Smooky helped me get to the next level, but each time I saw my Dancer, it broke my heart.

As spring was moving toward summer, I noticed that the Heubecks didn't come down to the barn as often to check on their horses at night, or even in the mornings. I knew something wasn't right. I thought that maybe the cold was keeping them away. One night Mr. Heubeck paid what had become a rare visit to the barn, and we sat down on a little wooden bench to talk.

"Where's Mrs. H at tonight?" I asked him with a smile.

"Oh," he said, sadly. "She's not going to be coming down as much anymore. They found a spot on her liver."

Although Mr. Heubeck tried to hide his pain, I could hear it in his voice, see it in the sag of his head. I reached over and put my callused hand over his worn one. This giant in the horse business burst into quiet tears, and I sat next to him, patting his hand. When he stood to walk back to the house, he could barely move. It was the only thing worse than saying he couldn't have horses anymore: his wife was leaving him.

The few times I saw Mrs. H, her stomach was distended and her skin was a sickly yellow color. Mr. Heubeck started coming down less and less to the barn—and then not at all. I knew she was dying. Then one day a fancy sports car was parked in their main driveway.

The Heubecks had a son who hadn't spoken to either of them in years because he had married a Korean woman, and they didn't approve. I saw a crumpled Mr. Heubeck on his front porch with his son, and I knew this loving, proud man couldn't handle the future by himself and had called for help. One day, while Mrs. H rested in their bedroom, Mr. Heubeck walked outside, but he didn't make it to the horses. He had a massive heart attack.

Mr. H had already had a bad heart, but he still got up on his horses every morning against doctor's orders. A decade passed without any trouble until that massive heart attack, which left him bedridden for several days at the farm until he passed away in his sleep.

I think his wife's illness killed him because he loved her so much, so different from my own father's response to my mother's sickness. They had a love I had imagined but never experienced. It was a rare gift they had that could only be shared together. Six weeks later, Mrs. H passed away.

They were gone, and I knew my time at Quail Roost II would soon be over. The fate of the farm was unsure, and no one there ever believed in me the way Mr. Heubeck had. Still, something had been given to me at this place, and I knew it could never be taken away. What I learned at the Heubeck's farm is that there are truly sincere people in this world who will open a door and their hearts to you, no matter what you look like or what ailment you have. The Heubecks inspired and motivated me to search for something higher than myself. Whenever I'm down, that unconditional love they showed me pulls me through.

Furlong Nine

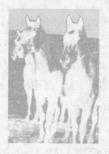

*N*ow I let Pegasus go. We pull away from the other mounts, and they steadily fall back, as if swallowed by the track. All but one, an upstart brown Thoroughbred with a look of intensity in his eyes. He certainly wasn't going to lose tonight—not to a horse that no one thought had a chance and a rider who was written off many years ago. But I think otherwise.

We ride neck and neck, but I almost want to laugh. There can be no stopping us now, me and Pegasus. I have wandered through too many valleys, stumbled across too many obstacles to be here. No one wants this race more than we do.

Breezing
Ocala, Florida

I felt a bit lost after losing the Heubecks. Questions of what to do next flooded my brain, and there were no easy answers. I could hear Mr. Heubeck's voice ringing in my ears: "Don't go to the track. Don't take your love of horses to the track. You don't really want to ride that way."

But I wanted to go fast and then faster. Mr. Heubeck knew that when he asked me to take two horses out together and breeze them. Breezing readies a horse for a race by building up wind speed by filling their lungs with more air. It's like a track runner. You might jog two miles, but as your sprints come up, you do quicker runs to get more power in your legs and air in your lungs. When breezing two horses, one gallops beside you like in a race. Mr. Heubeck might have been saying no to me racing, but in his own way he was preparing me to race. He knew what I wanted to do. *He knew.*

He also knew something I learned quickly: horse racing is a rough industry, and an even rougher life for those who choose it. Alcoholism and substance abuse counselors on every track in America could write a book on the challenges of living on the backstretch. In fact, some of them have. The pay isn't the best, and many of the people involved in the daily world of racing barely make a living. They often drown their sorrows in drugs and alcohol. Furthermore, the sport is dominated by men, many from foreign countries, with their own unique customs and biases against women as jockeys. Still, as with most concerns of passion, the reality of it doesn't matter. You try because you have to, because it is a part of you. In addition, I find some semblance of calm with horses. Interacting with them helps to keep me level. They are the reins that keep my madness in check.

Mr. Heubeck's farm was a safe, protected environment; unlike the harsh racetrack world I so craved. But I felt ready for it. My relationship with Mr. Heubeck had fortified me, and I didn't feel it was a coincidence that I had the chance to learn from him before he left this earth.

In my lingering days, as the Heubeck's farm was marked SOLD in big black letters across the real estate signs, I knew I had to find a place to live. But something else was pressing even harder inside me. I needed to know everything I could about training horses. If Mr. Heubeck couldn't mentor me anymore, then I would just have to mentor myself.

It was horse-breaking season, and in the local newspaper I found want ads asking for workers who knew how to start horses. I wondered, Am I good enough? I'm mostly self-taught—how will I stack up to the competition? Trainers from all over the world came to Florida in the winter to start horses. But I finally got my nerve up and decided to give it a try. I picked the Scanlon Farm, owned by an Irish family. I thought it was a good omen. My children Shauna and Ryan are half Irish. They are like my good-luck charms.

Robert Scanlon had a reputation, not just in this country but over the entire world, as a top-notch horseman. The royal family of Dubai bought the best horses in the world, ones that cost

$500,000 on upward. They kept sixty horses with Scanlon every year. There were million-dollar horses on this farm, which I would've found intimidating if I hadn't been blissfully unaware of price tags at the time.

When Mr. Scanlon chose people to take care of his horses, he needed to know that the horses were their first priority. I went to his farm and simply asked him for a job, providing a disclaimer: "I've only been riding a little bit of time, and I've started just a few babies."

He smiled, and I couldn't help suspecting that Mr. Heubeck might have mentioned me to him.

"Sylvia, why don't you just hang out here? Learn. Watch the other riders," he said.

It wasn't a job, but I was grateful, and I did as he suggested. The riders had on fine four-hundred-dollar boots and beautiful brand-new chaps. I was wearing my forty-dollar boots and had my old helmet and vest in the car—just in case. Don't get intimidated, I told myself; just talk to the people and watch. I didn't want to act like I was scared, even though I was.

While I observed, Mr. Scanlon had already decided he was going to give me a job. But first came a test. "Why don't you take this horse?" he said later in the day, handing me the reins of a gorgeous gray champion. "Back him up to the five-eighths pole. Then gallop a mile and a half."

I was excited. I knew what backing the horse up meant. I had done that plenty of times. I would ride the horse at a walk on the outside of the track, counter to the direction in which they would race. The pole was a marker for each furlong. But I didn't know the poles; we didn't use them at the Heubeck farm. Oh, my God, I thought. I'm going to blow this. But I stayed quiet, and acted like I knew what I was doing.

Hoisting myself onto the horse, I whispered to one of the hands, "Could you please point out the five-eighths pole?" He whispered to me that on the track the pole was around to the left. The eight-eighths pole is the mile pole, and then you go counterclockwise around the track—8, 7, 6, 5, and so on. At 5, you turn the horse around and start your gallop. I followed his directions and still couldn't find the pole. I went back to ask again, but he was gone.

I let out a nervous laugh. All of this doggone math, I thought. I couldn't even remember my fractions when I was in the fourth grade. If I messed this up, then I was gone from this gorgeous farm forever. Confused, I asked one of the riders to *please* point to the five-eighths pole, and he just looked me hard in the eyes and said nothing. I asked the next rider. He wouldn't talk either. The third looked at me with pity and trotted on. The fourth said, "Obviously, you're not supposed to be here jaw jacking with these types of horses." That encouraged me. I had nothing to lose, so I started jogging my horse clockwise back to the poles, where I encountered another rider who was next to me. I asked him—no, *pleaded* with him—to show me the five-eighths pole.

"Could you just tell me where it is?" I implored. "I've never done this before and I don't want to—"

"Yeah, yeah, yeah, I'll show you," he said with an eye roll.

So I took my gorgeous gray horse and followed this rider to the five-eighths pole. When I got there, I turned my horse around and did a nice gallop around the rest of the track. We were doing fine until two horses came out of nowhere and ran us into the rail. My horse didn't get hurt, but took off in a dead run. We were suddenly running across the track and into the grassy middle.

Damn it, damn it! I cried inside, finally getting control of the horse and making him come down to a slow trot.

"Well, there goes that," I said to no one in particular.

When I brought the horse back, I didn't say anything, and Mr. Scanlon didn't say anything, while a hand took the half-million-dollar baby inside the barn for a cooldown before going back into his stall. I was standing there awaiting the inevitable when Mr. Scanlon said, "Well, Sylvia, I'm going to give you a second shot. Make sure this time you don't let the horse run off, because this one is just back in the action from a knee injury."

Oh, man, I thought. If this one hurts himself, if he breaks his knee, I'm not only gone, I'll be sued. Suddenly I remembered Mr. Heubeck's words: "When you're galloping, always look like a monkey having sex with a football on the horse."

So that's what I did when I got on my new mount: looked like a monkey having sex with a football. Slowly but surely, I stayed way on the outside so nobody would make my horse run off—and it worked beautifully. When I came back to the barn, Mr. Scanlon said, "Have someone show Sylvia the baby barn."

One of the grooms materialized in two seconds and said, "Miss Sylvia, come with me. I'll show you the ten you'll be starting."

I enjoyed working at the Scanlon farm with all their majestic horses, but the job only lasted about six weeks. One day I saw a bunch of new riders in the paddock. They had arrived from up north and were obviously quite experienced with horses. Mr. Scanlon told me that it was their turn, and he would have to let me go.

"Don't give up," he said. "You're doing a great job. But I have enough people now, and I promised them jobs months ago. I'll give you the best reference."

Disappointed, I smiled at him and said, "Thank you for giving me a shot."

I needed work. I'd heard there was work at Sweetwater Stables, where they'd hire anybody for one hundred a day.

"Theresa will take care of you," I heard. "She'll even give you an extra fifty dollars now and then if she likes you. If she doesn't like you, then you get nothing."

I went to her farm, and she hired me on the spot. It was an intimidating place run by one tough horsewoman. Theresa, the owner, had black hair down past her rear end. She was an Italian from Boston, and I liked her because she had the reputation of being so tough. She was quite the character.

"Get your fucking ass in that stall and get your damn shit out of there right now," she shouted at one of the hands. Yes, she was vulgar, but I didn't see anyone opening up a mouth to her. She had nice horses, but not as superior as the Scanlons'. Yet her breeds still had a pedigree. She also had a lot of mares that popped out a lot of babies. I knew that Theresa would fire me on the spot if I messed up, yet I couldn't help it that her babies would sneak through the broken fence and get lost for a little bit. Yes, I lost (and found) them, but she never fired me, got mad, or even hollered at me.

Theresa continued to teach me and told me that she had wanted to be a horse jockey and had the petite build to do it, but she'd broken her back riding on her own farm. Her horse racing days weren't going to happen, but she wasn't a jealous woman if she saw someone who still could reach that finish line.

"Get on this one," Theresa said, putting me on top of some of her toughest horses. "No stick. No whip. This is between you and the horse." I loved that she wouldn't use a stick. So many riders were stick-happy.

She would say, "Don't you see a difference? Look at these fillies. You will end up on the ground nine times out of ten with the stick. Do it with your hands, Sylvia," she instructed, and she taught me how to touch a horse, to make it respond with firm kindness.

She put me on a beautiful gray Thoroughbred baby, from the direct line of the famed horse Storm Cat, a grandson of Kentucky Derby winner Northern Dancer and Triple Crown champion Secretariat. We had already met each other in the stall and paddock area, but we hadn't been to the track yet. This baby was a bit ornery, but he allowed me to put him through his paces with my hands guiding him around the track.

In the mornings Theresa would clean all the stalls herself, which was unheard of for a woman in her position. She was an owner and a stall cleaner? I learned that she had cancer and just wanted to be around the horses for as long as possible. Theresa made a few bad calls, including hiring a smart-ass rider named Billy who drank and did crack and speed when no one was looking. I was the only female and the smallest rider, so Billy took particular pleasure in goading me.

One day I was riding on Storm Cat baby, he came up very close behind me with his horse. You don't bum-rush someone who is walking their horse peacefully by running up next to them. Nine times out of ten the rider who is walking will get thrown. Thanks to Billy, the baby bolted up on his hind legs and dumped me.

"Oh, sorry," Billy said. "I certainly didn't mean to do it."

"If you don't care about my life, maybe you could think about this baby horse breaking its legs," I warned, but he didn't care.

Meanwhile, I found another little pony for sale. For $2,500, I could have another Medicine Hat. This one had a big cute mole right on his nose. I couldn't resist him and ripped my savings out of the bank to buy and then board him. Meanwhile, the broken-down Thoroughbred that I'd traded Dancer for was now clean, healthy, groomed, and ready to go to a racetrack, which was thrilling for me. I was searching for a trainer and knew it was just a matter of time before my own horse would be racing.

In the midst of this horse nirvana, I got a call from my mother. It was the first in a long time. We had not spoken much since Mioshi was burned. Over time I'd mellowed out, and Mioshi had begun to flourish; he was a grade ahead of where he was supposed to be in school. I talked to him often. He had even calmed down due to his injuries, and perhaps learned a lesson from them. The permanent scarring served as a reminder of the dangers of playing with fire and, more important, that I wasn't there. That I had failed as his mom.

My father continued to raise Mioshi, and as time passed, my son healed. My relationship with my father was healing too. But I was a little more wary of my mother. She could be difficult for me to deal with. Although I didn't doubt her love for me, she could be harsh and judgmental.

"Sylvia, I think I'm going to move out your way," she told me.

It was as if a bomb had dropped through the phone lines. I felt I was finally getting my life together. My horse was ready for the track, plus I had a cute little apartment. I still missed the TLC from the Heubecks, but I had a few friends at my job who provided laughs and a friendly ear. The new pony, which I purchased even though I should have saved the money, had promise, and Theresa was my new mentor. The last thing I was looking for was any emotional upsets. I hadn't had a serious episode since I immersed myself in the horses, but I didn't know if I was strong enough to handle the stress of having my mother, who herself was quite needy, living with me.

Still, for whatever reason, I could never say no to my mother. She arrived the next week and moved in with me. Late that first night, she told me she had grown lonely in California and worried about me. It was an unexpected moment, and I thought maybe it could be a new beginning for the two of us. I was wrong.

Daily, I was up at 5:30 to begin my day with Theresa. I knew my mother was still ill, but I had two horses, a job with more horses, and the pressure of earning a living. I couldn't stop to take care of my mother, but I suspected that was the real reason she'd decided to come live with me.

From the minute we drove in from the airport and my mother saw the big black iron gates outside my new apartment, I knew we were going to clash.

"Wow, this is an expensive place," she said. She sounded surprised and somehow disapproving. She hounded me about everything. First, it was about the groceries. I didn't have enough.

"I gotta go to work, Mom," I said early the next day. "When I come back, we can go out and get groceries." She insisted we go when she wanted. And like a good daughter, I obliged her.

After work that night, for the first time in a long time, I felt like a nervous wreck.

The day after that, I took her on a tour of the farm and showed her the horses I was working with. My mother has never been a real animal person. She loves dogs and cats, but she's not horse crazy. She never bothered to ask which horse was mine or if I planned to race. "It's getting late, Mom, and I have to get up early to feed the horses," I said with a sigh. "Let's just go home."

She kept picking at me in a way that only moms can do. One night over dinner, my mother told me a story about a family member who had been burned beyond recognition. "Have you ever looked at the scars of a burn victim, Sylvia?" she asked me. She wasn't talking about my son, but it triggered me. Did she know what she was saying? Was she trying to taunt me? Or was she speaking, as she often did, without thinking?

"As a matter of fact, Mom," I said, "no, I didn't get the opportunity to see my son with his skin burned off."

"Don't start that with me," my mother warned.

"I got too much going on to start," I warned her.

"Get off your high horse, Sylvia," my mother said. "You think you're this and that now. But I'm here to remind you who you really are—just plain Sylvia."

This is not going to get to me, I thought, closing my eyes. She is not going to get to me. But the truth is, members of my family upset me in a way no others can. I tried to remain calm, level, but I could feel tension starting to wind its way through me. I had to do something.

I had always wanted to buy my mother a house, and I thought that this might be the time to try and do so. She was thrilled at the idea. I looked around for a little rent-to-own house, which seemed like the perfect solution. I found one in Ocala by the farms and near my horses. Three bedrooms would be enough space for my mom and me to keep out of each other's hair—or so I thought.

The owner wanted $2,500 down, and I didn't have all the money. My mom called my grandmother, who was always very abusive toward my mother, which probably explains the tension that we feel at times. It was a miracle that my grandmother sent us the money. We put a down payment on our new house together, with me trying to make the monthly payments. The rent was seven hundred a month, and I had to ride and train consistently to afford this sharp increase in living expenses.

From the start, my mother wasn't content with the new house. Decorating a new place didn't consume her, and she still insisted on calling me all day long. My time was filled with her needing this and that, and the demands were constant. One day she casually announced, "I might need to go back to the hospital for my stomach." As I rushed around, getting everything in order, she changed her mind and decided she didn't want to go anywhere.

Another time she called my cell phone while I was galloping. "Sylvia, I need to go to the doctor. I need my meds," she cried.

"I can't go now, Mom," I told her. "You need to have the elderly care bus pick you up."

"No, now," she said. "Come home right now."

"Mom," I said, "I have to work, and my horses need to be cleaned and fed. This is my life. This is my day. I didn't know you were coming here needing all of this care. I'm trying to be compassionate, but—"

Forcing myself to shut my mouth, I took a breath; I knew my mother wasn't well. She wasn't happy, and the Buddhist in me knew I had to change the karma. For the first time in a long time, I was fearful of relapsing into a place I didn't trust.

My mother continued to ride me daily. The more she picked, the more nervous I got, and that led to a few accidents on the horses. There is no way in the world that this is a coincidence, I thought. She also called me several times a day with "emergencies"—like, she needed cigarettes immediately.

"I have horses that need to eat," I told her. "Cigarettes can wait."

It was all upsetting, and the tension was excruciating. Slowly but surely, I fell off more horses and found myself on the ground, literally and later figuratively. I couldn't seem to focus, and I felt short-tempered more and more often. Perhaps it wouldn't have been so difficult with my mom if we hadn't been estranged for such a long time. But I had issues, and she continued, sometimes unintentionally, to push my buttons. I'd never forgiven her for not telling me about my son's burns. In my heart, I knew that someday Mioshi in turn would blame me for not being there as his mother. But I hadn't been allowed to be there.

Resentment and distance made living with my mother impossible. It galled me that all of a sudden she wanted to pretend that nothing had happened between us. My horses were becoming more important to me than my mother; I needed them. I still tried to do as much as I could, but deep down I knew it wasn't going to work. I'm not the same person around my family. There's just too much baggage. No matter what I do, I'm always Sylvia, the crazy one.

My inner self had begun to percolate, and my moods began to rush. It wasn't as bad as before, but I knew the longer I stayed with my mother, the greater the chances that I would be driven to an institution like Western. Feeling manic and unstable, I still went about my daily routine, picking up hay and feed for the horses, hoping that could take the place of medication and its side effects. One day I was turning into the local feed store when, *bam!* a truck rear-ended me, and I was almost thrown through the windshield. The impact tore up my new Volvo, and then in the confusion another car bashed into the side of mine when that same truck sideswiped it. Bruised and aching, I went home to find little sympathy from my mother.

"Why do these things always happen to you?" she asked impatiently. I went to my room and closed the door.

My mania surfaced at work, and Theresa was starting to show her frustration with me. I couldn't stay focused. You have to be alert around horses at all times. And I wasn't. I was full-blown manic. I tried to hide it as much as I could, but without medication and with the pressure I felt from my mom, I was falling apart at the seams.

"Either you're going to get killed, or a horse is going to be seriously hurt," Theresa said one day. Then, as I had expected, she let me go. Not long after, I lost all my jobs because I couldn't focus on any of them. In the blink of an eye, everything I'd built so slowly was falling apart. I couldn't even handle my own racehorse, and he was ready to go to the track. My beautiful life in Florida was trickling away.

In the midst of my despair, Mother packed up one day and announced that she was going back to California. Maybe she thought it would be easier on me financially if she wasn't there; she never said. But like a sudden summer storm that sweeps out to sea, leaving destruction in its path, she was gone.

I was conflicted. On the one hand, with her gone, perhaps there would be less of a trigger for my emotions. But at the same time, with everything falling apart again, I felt abandoned. Unable to pay the rent, I lost the new house and found myself back in a trailer, with no money to pay for my life. I could just barely make enough to pay for my two horses with a lackluster job at a lesser horse farm.

One day I picked up a *Thoroughbred Times* and saw an ad for a company accepting racehorses. It seemed like an amazing deal. I didn't have to pay any bills; they would get my horse ready to race, and we would split the winnings. It was perfect timing. My horse was ready to go to the track. He needed to get on with his life, but I didn't have any money to spend on a horse trailer now.

This company was the solution.

After chanting and praying, I called the number on the ad and talked to a very sweet woman, who told me about her love of racehorses. "I know he's special," I told her.

"He sounds like an amazing horse," said the woman. "All we need to do is for you to put the horse into our hands. We'll move him to our location and then split his winnings."

"What do I have to pay?" I asked.

"We pay his food and board," she said. "You pay some of his day rates for racing. When he wins, we split the profits." She gave me the number of the trainer who would be working with my horse, and we talked for a long time. She was a compassionate person who knew horses, so I felt comfortable with her.

The toughest part was paying for a horse trailer to take my horse to West Virginia, where this company was based. A ride to West Virginia from Florida cost around $410 one way, and I didn't have an extra dime to my name—not to mention that I'd ruined my credit with the last rent-to-own disaster. All I had was this run-down trailer I was living in with my dog and a stray cat I had taken in.

It was the end of April 2004, and my racehorse was my only salvation. I never bet money on a horse in my life because I don't believe in betting; I'm superstitious about it. But it was Kentucky Derby time, and I scrounged around and found $112, which was all I had to my name. I placed a bet locally, and a jockey friend of mine laughed when I put my money down.

"You're going to lose your ass on that order of horses," he promised.

But I bet my last dime on getting enough cash together to send my beloved Thoroughbred, Smooky, to West Virginia to start his career. Lo and behold, I hit a trifecta and a superfecta, which totaled $440. Yes, that meant I had thirty dollars extra to buy my Smooky a little food once he got to his new training grounds up north.

I called a horse van company and brought Smooky for transport. It was strange that on the day he was to leave, my horse resisted. He was an animal that always listened to me, but this time he was refusing to get in that trailer. Smooky didn't "load up good," as they say in the horse business. In fact, we had to back him in, ass forward, to get him to leave.

I was walking him and thinking, "Why are you being such a handful?" Once he was in the van, the horse refused to look at me. Smooky knew it was time to go; he knew we were saying good-bye.

The trainer in West Virginia accepted shipment of my horse, but as time passed, she cut off contact with me and disappeared with my Smooky. I began to worry that I had been hustled. I even went to the sheriff's office, but there was nothing much they could do for me. And without much in the way of resources, there wasn't anything I could do.

I was a wreck, and my sadness was palpable. Things hadn't worked out with my mom, my job was gone, and I'd lost my horse and my house. I was in a fast spiral downward, but still working with horses. My manic energy continued to appear, but it was mixed with such sadness that the manic highs were met with true lows. It would take a lot for me to get back into a good space again. I started to wonder if it was even worth it to try.

Theresa heard my sad story and hired me back on at her farm, but I wasn't riding with the same enthusiasm. At night the trailer park was like one large drug den, and I tried to hide out with my doors tightly locked. All night long, people who were flying high on crack would bang on my door, screaming, "You got two dollars? You got a cigarette?"

I just closed my eyes until they went away. Then the bad

dreams would come, of Smooky and what had happened to him. What had they done with my beautiful horse? Did they hurt him? Were they mistreating him? There was nobody to help me get him back.

A couple of months later, I drove up to West Virginia on a tip that someone had seen Smooky with these new people. I found the horse and these thieves, who now told me I owed them thousands of dollars for his board and feed. Meanwhile, the trainer told me he was "legged up" and good enough to run. "You did an excellent job with him," she said. "But now he belongs to us. If you try to take him, we'll call the police."

I patted Smooky on the nose, and he nuzzled me. When I started to walk off, he followed in a desperate plea to get away. If I could have jumped on his back and rode him away, I would have. But they would have certainly stopped me. They claimed that I'd given them ownership in the horse, and they had rights. I wanted to fight them legally, but with what?

That horse taught me to gallop and ride. My heart broke for him, and I was tired. I went back to Florida to let go of my other horse. I sold him, and that helped. But my money was low. I moved around from farm to farm, looking for work without much success. I rarely feel the other pole of my illness, the one that makes you lie in bed underneath covers and sleep for hours and hours. It's not as exhilarating and creative as the highs. But this time I was low. Depressed, I left Florida and returned to my father and son in Virginia. I went home.

Furlong Ten

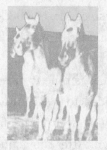

We pass the final pole, and my heart starts pounding louder than a bass drum, not from fear but from excitement. We are so close to the finish I can feel it, and yet it still seems so far away. The brown Thoroughbred is beside us, determined to rupture my fairy-tale ending. This is it. You've got to go all out and push yourself and the horse. That final stretch determines if you are a finisher or a winner.

Arlington Park and Hawthorne Race Course
Chicago and Cicero, Illinois

I went home and rested. It was a good time. Mioshi, Dad, and I got along. We enjoyed each other's company. I was Mom again. Fixing my son's breakfast, dropping him off at school, and being there for him when he went to sleep at night made me feel so lucky. I was also reconnecting with my dad, who seemed to get it that I really wanted to be a jockey. The more I explained the horse racing business to him, the more he understood my passion about it. That helped me tap into a sense of empowerment that had been missing since Mr. Heubeck died.

But I was getting anxious. It wasn't the mania. I was missing the horses.

It was May 2005. It was time to ride again. I couldn't really leave the game. I decided to head up to Canada to find some work with horses, having seen an ad for a jockey at Marquis Downs in Saskatchewan. After contacting a sponsor, who promised he was excited to meet me and would file the papers I needed to work in Canada, I packed up what little I had, said good-bye to Dad and Mioshi, and left Virginia.

When I reached the border at North Portal, North Dakota, I learned that I hadn't filed the necessary papers I needed to work in Canada. I would have to go to the Canadian consulate in Detroit and pay three to five thousand dollars for a work visa. I had eighty dollars in my pocket. More than anything, I couldn't stand telling my father that I was stuck again and needed money. But I had no choice. I'd have to go back to Staunton.

While still in North Portal, I went to a library to find the closest Buddhist temple. When all else fails, I continue to chant and pray. At first, I looked for a temple in North Portal, and then I started looking for temples in cities near racetracks just for the hell of it. I saw that Chicago had a temple and a track that were close to each other. I checked my stash. I didn't have enough gas money to make it back to Virginia or Florida. Chicago was the closest option. My choice was made for me.

I drove straight to the temple, which was located in the Chicago suburbs. Exhausted and dejected, I was welcomed at the temple by a woman who greeted me with open arms. She asked a little bit about my life. When I told her about my love of horses, she smiled and said, "Did you know that the Arlington Park racetrack is only twenty minutes from here? It's one of the most gorgeous places in the area."

Arlington Park is located in the upper-middle-class suburb of Arlington Heights, Illinois, about a forty-five-minute drive outside of Chicago. Nearly a decade ago, the track caught on fire and the entire place burned to the ground in a massive inferno. This racing palace was rebuilt bigger than ever, and from the road it shone white in the early-morning sunshine, reminding me of a temple. It was morning, and the horses were being put through their paces. This place is breathtaking, I thought as I swung my car around in the lot to get a view of the gorgeous horses that were in various stages of training. From my years in Florida, I knew what to do next. Locking the car, I walked inside and went from barn to barn, asking if anyone needed a trained worker who could breeze or gallop or even muck the stalls. An owner hired me to exercise three of her horses—that is, to gallop them—and I went back to my car with $50.

I also learned that the tracks in Chicago were among the most competitive in the nation and wouldn't exactly greet an almost-forty female jockey with much enthusiasm.

"You want to be a jock?" one of the trainers said in an amazed voice. "Good luck getting mounts. Plus you'll need your license, which might take a long time."

I mulled it over as I got a room for the night, but no food; my budget didn't allow for both eating and sleeping. I was back to those days. The next morning, hungry but excited, I went back to Arlington and rode a few more horses for another $50. I went back each and every day, and learned that I could earn $100 or $120 for exercising horses, and I could go to that wonderful temple each night to pray.

It was warm outside, so I took again to living in my car near the track. Staying in the backside dorms at Arlington wasn't an option for exercise riders. But it didn't matter; I was excited to be at this place. Suddenly I was a new face, known for having a good set of hands and excellent horse sense, though my horse sense was not the norm.

"Use your stick to make the horse move," a trainer told me.

"I don't take directions from people when I'm on a horse; I take directions from the horse," I responded.

"What?"

"I've never met a person as smart as a horse," I concluded, wondering how a man who weighed three hundred pounds and had never been on the back of a horse could tell me what to do. And why would he want to tell me that, when the horse was responding perfectly with no stick?

Fabulous horses surrounded me at Arlington Park, and I quickly figured out that it wasn't the horses' fault if they didn't perform; it was the people they were around. I worked for many of the trainers on a rotating basis—some good, some bad, but each taught me something.

One day I got on top of It's No Joke, a horse that won the Hawthorne Gold Cup that year. I felt like I was on the back of a cloud when we sailed around the expansive cushioned track. He was a big, gentle baby, and I couldn't even feel his feet touch the ground. The first time I sat on him, he turned around and looked me right in the eye. He must have liked what he saw, because suddenly we were off for our ride through the stratosphere.

I wasn't sure I would ever be a jockey, but in the way I had come to make decisions, sometimes suddenly, always intuitively, it became increasingly important for me to get my jock's license. I figured I had just as much a right as anyone else to apply for a jockey's license, although there were times that I thought I might quit this dream, it seemed so ridiculous.

"Why would you quit now?" one of the trainers, who was also my friend, demanded. "All you need is the money and to ride a couple of times to get your approval mounts for your license."

I knew that for the most part, he was right. I would have to apply and get approval from the stewards, who are the officials for the track. In addition, the head outrider who leads the horses to the gate for each race would also have to give his approval. They would all have to see me ride a number of times to prove that I knew all the rules of the racetrack and that I posed no danger to myself or other riders.

They didn't know about my condition, and I made sure not to mention it. If I did anything crazy, I hoped it would be attributable to the characteristics of the many players in the horse world, not because I was "different." And if all went well, I could get my apprentice jockey license after riding two approval mounts in two races. At some tracks, you were required to have five approval mounts for your license, but at Arlington it was only two.

I worked steadily, exercising and grooming horses, and in the process began to develop a rapport with many of the trainers. It was hard work, and I didn't know if anyone would take me seriously, but still, being around the horses and focusing on them calmed me. I felt it was the best therapy I could have. Then one day in August, I was given the chance to ride in my first professional race.

My heart was beating wildly as I put on the equipment I had bought with my earnings and mounted a horse in the blazing noon sunshine of a midwestern summer. "Go out there and have a nice ride," said Manny, a trainer who helped me to the starting gate for my first time as a jockey. As I waited at the starting gate for the bell, all of it came flooding back to me: my father leaving, the manic episodes, losing my children, going to California, losing my Mioshi, his being burned, my rebirth in Ocala with the horses. *Yes, all those glorious horses.*

I kept saying, "And look where I am now!"

I chanted *Nam-myoho-renge-kyo* silently to myself and grabbed my horse's mane as the bell sounded. And we were off! It didn't matter that my horse was old, or that we were thirty lengths behind the other horses. I knew I didn't look so good, but I was still out there—as a racehorse jockey.

Afterward, I was on a high that lasted for a week. All I needed was one more approval mount before I could get my license. Nobody seemed to have a horse for me to ride in a race, and that played on my mind. I was okay to ride and breeze their horses. I could gallop and exercise them for the other jockeys. But no one seemed to think I was good enough to race.

At the same time, a pretty young blond woman came to the track, who also wanted to be a jockey. Of course, there were plenty of mounts for a girl that all the owners and trainers wanted to date. Manny came to my rescue and said he would certainly find me a second mount that week. He kept his word, and I placed fifth on the mount he got me, which was actually pretty good for a rider with no license, on a horse with no future. This brown Thoroughbred hadn't run in over a year and had a bad knee, but his performance on the track earned me my jockey's license.

Tom Morgan, a jockey agent, actually called the *Chicago Sun-Times* about me. He has a friend who's a sportswriter, and this was what Tom called some story. "She's middle aged, black, and wants to be a jockey," he said. "It's a helluva story."

Apparently it was, because the paper ran a nice tidbit, which was a big deal for me.

At first I didn't tell anyone, not even my family, about my jockey's license. The first thing I knew I would hear was, "You're too old. You're too poor. You're too done." There had been so much discouragement in my life, I didn't want to set myself up for ridicule. Yet I started thinking. I knew I was almost forty; I knew I was poor; I knew I might even be done; but I *did* have my license. I knew I might not ever be a great jockey, but *I got to be a jockey.* Never again would someone be able to tell me that I couldn't do something.

Being homeless, black, female, and middle-aged hadn't stopped me. Physical and emotional abuse didn't keep me from my moment. Despite the stays in mental hospitals and my ongoing struggle with being bipolar, I was now a jockey. In a strange way, the illness helped me pursue this course, as dealing with horses had proved more effective than meds for keeping me level. That was good, since the cost factor as well as issues with side effects were a big deterrent to taking my meds.

The racing circuit moves from track to track, and it was time to leave Arlington. I decided to try Hawthorne Race Course in Cicero. It was a more raggedy track than Arlington, but I had heard that I would do better over there as a jockey. "You won't get many mounts at Arlington," Manny told me. "But you'll get some at Hawthorne."

Horse racing is such a male-dominated sport that, as a woman, I couldn't get many mounts. I just had to stick it out and look for opportunities, then hope I might get lucky. At Hawthorne I could get mounts, but they were always old or injured; the ones nobody wanted to ride. When I was offered a half decent horse, a more experienced jockey would always try to talk the owner out of it and say, "Oh, you're going to put her on it? She's real green. I'll take it now instead."

There was no way to win or even place on a horse that had been out twenty times but never won one race. These horses are broken down. On the track we will say, "That horse is a nickel." That's about all the horse is worth. The owners still look at a lost race on a nickel as if it's the jockey's fault; everyone looks at it that way. The horse isn't a loser; you are.

Weeks went by at Hawthorne where nobody had a horse for

me. I so longed for Mr. Heubeck's influence. Instead, the closest I came was with a family of owners called the Haysticks, who were ruled off the track at Hawthorne because their horses weren't taken care of in the right manner. It wasn't that they were lazy; this family struggled financially. We always liked each other, and I rode their horses for exercise. They owed me money and couldn't pay, but I still went back to them to see if they needed help. This family was a group of outcasts on the track, and I identified with that.

One day the Haysticks called me over to ask if I wanted a mount for an afternoon race. I knew their horse was too old to win. They didn't have the money, so their horse wasn't going to be one hundred percent prepared. But I had a soft spot for their daughter, who was so sweet and said, "I want you to race my horse, Miss Sylvia. You can make him win. He loves you."

I knew if this horse didn't win, I'd be blamed by the wife, who got a little riled with the jocks who didn't pull off miracles. I'm still making money galloping in the morning, I thought, trying to console myself. Even if I mess up as a jock, there is always a backup plan. We rode that afternoon, not for money or glory but for the love of the sport. In a Hollywood movie, I would've come in first as some grand music played in the background. But this was the real world. I came in dead last.

There's a misconception that the minute you get on a horse as a jockey, you're suddenly making major dough. I was on those mounts for about $45 a ride, risking life and limb trying to win a horse race at Hawthorne. It's a dangerous sport; you're in a pack of horses going so fast that one wrong move could mean a broken neck or severed spinal cord.

I didn't focus on that extreme, but rather the embarrassment of not looking good in a race. If you're losing on a horse, and that animal doesn't really even have the energy to finish, then people, including owners and trainers, say, "Oh, I told you she couldn't ride." Most of my mounts were with the worst, most broken-down horses, horses that didn't have the pep for a brisk walk around the track, let alone a race.

The catch-22 is that if you keep losing, no one wants to give you mounts, but you can't get mounts unless you race on something. You can't learn how to race unless you're out there in the heart of the pack, pounding your way toward the finish line.

I wanted so badly to prove that I could do it, because I knew I could.

"But you can't win, so don't even think about it," a trainer told me. "It takes years to win a horse race."

A big part of me wanted to quit. I had accomplished my goals, which were to get my license as a jockey and ride in a professional race. At the same time, what was I to do if somebody said, "Sylvia, I got one for you here. He's got bad legs, but you can try to make him win"?

So I kept at it, and it proved to be difficult. Even when I was galloping or breezing in the morning, it didn't mean I'd get a mount for the afternoon races. Most of the times the owners would have me breeze the horse and then pick a male jockey for the mount. Many didn't even pay me for the breezing, but considered it a favor and a way to decide if they would give me a mount.

"You have to give me the mount for me to breeze," I told one of the owners when we met at dawn on a freezing fall morning.

As dark rain clouds covered the sky, he said, "You got it. Now I really need you to get out there." After I did the breezing, he came back and said, "Maybe you're just not ready for a mount, but thanks for letting me take a look at you."

At night, I would sometimes talk to my mom on the phone.

"Where are you, Sylvia?" she asked. "Are you winning?"

I couldn't tell her that not only wasn't I winning, I mostly wasn't even riding in the races. I would simply say, I'm working on it, and tell her I would surely be in a race by December. She was excited for me. I was surprised and scared at the same time. I didn't want to disappoint her or me. I had to get some mounts. I worked harder than ever.

It wasn't easy. I got the worst of the worst. I breezed horses with fevers or internal problems, and ones that should have been left in the barn to heal. This is a brutal sport for man and horse. Pain on all levels is a given. I was on familiar terms with pain. But it was tough dealing with the other jocks, who didn't exactly welcome a black woman into their circle.

One day I came back to the jock's room, a large locker room filled with showers, benches, and areas to wait and dress before a race. Wandering over to my locker, I saw that someone had placed a KKK sign made with an old shower curtain by my locker.

"You need a pretty thick skin," one of the jocks told me with a smile. "The guys can be a little ruthless."

I could shrug off being passed over for a mount, but such an intentional obscenity threatened the precarious emotional balance I struggled for. I had been off my meds for a while, but staying balanced thanks to the horses. This, however, was extremely trying. I would chant for long periods and remind myself, I'm no good to anyone, not even the horses, if I'm sick. And then I got a break.

It was an early November day when trainer Charlie Bettis mentioned that he had a horse with arthritic knees named Wildwood Pegasus. No jockeys wanted to ride him because they feared his knees would collapse during a race, and both horse and rider could easily end up dead.

"Sylvia, I'd like you to get to know this horse. I promise that I will give you a mount," Charlie told me. I believed him and breezed Peg, which wasn't easy because of the horse's attitude. Charlie told me about how he had been hurt as a baby and felt wary of humans. He would even thrash around his stall all night long, an angry soul who was clearly dissatisfied with his circumstances. I would rub ointment on his legs every night the way Mr. Heubeck showed me to help with his knee.

A week later, Charlie offered me a mount on Peg.

"Do you think his leg will hold?" I asked, and Charlie nodded.

I caught the other jockeys giving my horse a look of disdain. They were none too pleased to be having a team they saw as a liability racing with them. The last thing they wanted was to be taken down by a collapsing mount. It was the last thing I wanted too. I kept talking to Peg as we rode up to the gate. I kept telling him we were going to be fine. I was trying to reassure myself as much as Peg. I think I was breathing harder than he.

When we took off, I could feel a surge of strength in him, and instead of lagging behind, we were in the front. It crossed my mind that the pace might be too much for his knee, but I put it out of my mind immediately. I didn't want him to sense my concern. When you're riding a horse, if you know what you're doing, you become a conduit for each other's emotions.

Peg was still going strong as we neared the home stretch— could we possibly win? There were four of us ahead of the rest. Concerned about his knee, I didn't want to push Peg. Still, he was holding his own. He pulled even with the lead horse, and my eyes must have gotten as big as the track. I could feel the finish line, but then the horse behind us made his move. I could tell from how he was coming, we wouldn't be able to hold him off. Then, in what seemed a flash, it was over. We didn't take first, but we did come in third.

Hot damn! Third! I was ecstatic. What's more, I knew Peg had it in him to win. I couldn't wait to tell my family. They were thrilled. A few days later, my mother called to let me know that Riley, Shauna, and Ryan were coming to the States for the holidays. Would I be racing? I explained to my mother that jockeys, especially "bugs" (as apprentice jockeys are called) like me, never know when they're going to race. She didn't care, she said. My entire family—Mom, Dad, Shauna, Riley, Ryan, my brother Ed Jr., and my baby Mioshi—wanted to see what I was doing, and they were coming to the track the first of December.

I was terrified. Of course, I was happy that my family was finally supporting me. But what if I tanked? What if I didn't even get a mount the day that they came? I tried not to think about it. But as the day of their arrival drew near, I knew that if I didn't stay focused on Pegasus, the family's visit could be a trigger for me.

Peg and I grew into our relationship during those cold nights, as winter got around to blasting the Midwest. The other trainers ignored the thrashing horse, so I stuck around to give him a good-night carrot or piece of apple. It reminded me of my days with Mr. Heubeck. And just like that white-haired old man, Peg slowly warmed up to me, and soon considered me to be his girl.

On the first of December, my family showed up as promised. But we didn't spend much time together. While they toured Chicago, I was in a zone. I didn't know if I'd have a mount or not, but I kept chanting, knowing that everything would fall into divine order. On my way to the track, the weatherman on the radio kept screaming about a major ice and sleet storm. I worried that the track might shut down, and my family would miss out on seeing any races, let alone one with me in it. When I got to the backside, Charlie told me, "Sylvia, jog Peg. He's riding tonight." He didn't mention who would be on his back, so I knew it wasn't me. This hurt, but I still took the opportunity to give my Peg a nice morning. I liked the way this formerly broken horse was riding with ease. The sky had already opened, and soft snow covered the track. In a strange way, this provided a nice cloudy cushion for a horse with an aching arthritic knee.

Later that afternoon, I was sitting in the jock's room, listening to who would get mounts that night for the first race of December. One horse was dubbed ill and unsafe to ride. One of the jocks said he didn't want to ride a different horse. And so it went, as the scrambling continued into the late-afternoon hours.

"How come Peg doesn't have a mount?" I announced, and heads turned my way, though usually I was just ignored or tormented. These men didn't have any time or patience for the lone woman in their presence. But I didn't care about their attitudes that night. *My family is here*, I thought. *I have to get a mount.*

"Why doesn't Peg have a jock on him?" I repeated.

"I don't know." That was the answer from the track manager.

"That horse is fine," I said. "I've been on him every morning, and he's better and better each day. Someone should ride him."

I don't know why, but I called Charlie and told him that Peg didn't have a rider. "I'll call Peg's owner," Charlie said. "If they say you can ride him tonight, Sylvia, will you?"

He knew the answer. Minutes later, I found out I was to ride Peg.

What should have been a wildly wonderful night started miserably. In the horse racing game, each rider is given a valet. A valet is necessary for a laundry list of reasons. He (they're mostly men) keeps your boots and your gear clean for you while also cleaning off your whip, if it's covered with sand and dirt after the races. He will help you tack up your horse for a race and put the saddle on. He basically does everything for a rider before a race, even bringing the rider his or her goggles before arriving at the starting line and some soap and a towel after it's all over.

My valet and I had a spat. He wasn't enthusiastic about being my valet and was doing a half-assed job, simply going through the motions and at a very slow speed—which I told him. He quit, much to the sneers and smiles of the other jocks, who knew I was up the creek without him. Although I should've been more diplomatic. It meant that I couldn't even get ready to ride Peg for the race. So many other valets and jocks were just standing around, shooting the bull, I was hoping one them would stand up and take his place. Silence was the only sound that permeated the jock's room when the jock's clerk shouted out, "Does anybody want to be Sylvia Harris's valet tonight?" But working for the one woman riding that night was the last thing they would ever do. They certainly weren't going to help some female who *thought* she could ride racehorses.

My race was forty-five minutes away, and this was an inopportune time for my valet to ditch me. I was shamed when nobody else stood up. For a split second, I thought that perhaps a personal appeal might help the situation.

"Come on, you guys. Can't someone help me? Please," I asked the valets who remained quiet.

Then I glanced at the clerk, who wouldn't even answer me anymore. With a shrug that indicated he was out of answers, he walked away, leaving me standing alone.

I didn't have my silks or my number, my girth or my saddle.

"I need some help," I implored as the other jocks just continued their conversations and routines as if no one was speaking.

"You guys," I finally cried out, "are a bunch of real jerks."

And with those words, I walked back into the jock room to gather myself and regroup so I wouldn't get thrown off my game The hotbox, or dry sauna, was waiting in the corner, and I stepped into it and closed the heavy wooden door behind me. It was the only place to find some nice solitude to do my prayers before the race.

When I stepped out of the hot box, I calmly announced, "I still need my silks. I need my equipment."

Again, my requests were met by disinterest and an almost childish silence. Finally, the clerk emerged again, and I told him if I had any more problems that night, there would be a major complaint filed with the owners of the track.

"I want my silks and my equipment without any more hassles," I said calmly.

From the back of the room, the clerk himself emerged with my stuff; it was not technically his job, but nobody else would do it. Dressing in silence for my race, I knew I had one more ritual to complete, which was to grasp my special jade prayer beads. I reached into my locker for my last dose of courage, my hands roaming the tiny shelves once . . . and then again. My precious beads were gone.

I always wore the beads somewhere on my body during every race, and I didn't have a spare set at the track. Obviously, the men had noticed the beads and were making another statement about how welcome I was in that jock's room. Instead of being crushed, I felt a strange, pure defiance sweeping into my blood, and I began to shift my mind-set. I convinced myself that the valet fiasco and the stolen beads were just a sign, but not one of devastation. I've survived far worse, knowing that obstacles are nothing but a sign of good things to come.

Instead of being angry, I found an empty stall, set up my makeshift alter, and chanted silently. I knew the childish antics of grown men weren't going to deter me from having the ride of my life.

The Finish

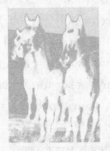

*O*tap Peg ever so slightly on the shoulder, and he pulls ahead. In both of our positions, there is one given: we have no more time to waste. The brown Thoroughbred begins to fade; he can only watch us as we pull farther away. We are flying. I recall the first time I ever saw a race. I was impressed with the magnificence of the horses. The power. I feel an exhilaration sweeping over me. Unlike the manic-driven cycles, this is real, organic to the moment. I am in the moment, and I am going to win!

Then, suddenly, Pegasus loses his footing.

In sickening slow motion, he pitches forward, lurching toward the frozen ground. All goes silent around me. My mind flashes back to the day before on the same track where there was a devastating accident during a race much like this one—a cold, snowy night with freezing sleet greeting both horse and rider. The light ice daggers falling from the sky at forty miles per hour were like a million tiny slaps to both athletes. Horses went down in horrendous spills during the race, and it was a miracle that their riders weren't killed. But two were seriously injured. One was a sixteen-year-old apprentice who was still in a coma, while the other rider was a veteran who busted himself up again for the umpteenth time. My mind can't help but play out the worst-case scenarios. But I cannot and will not give up.

"Come on, Peg, pull through it. We're not going down, not after all this." I doubt that he can hear me over the wind blowing and the harsh sound of his hoofs hitting the ice, but it doesn't matter. I'm sure he can feel what I feel: determination.

Peg pounds over the icy, frozen ground, legs upright and strong, and regains his balance as I shout encouragement. The upstart brown Thoroughbred is once again on us, having used our faltering to his advantage.

I tap Pegasus one last time, and he accelerates as if shot out of a cannon. It's all we need. We break away from the other horse, and ten feet from the finish line I am tempted to let go and extend my arms the way I did as a child atop my runaway horse, but I don't. I wait until I've crossed the finish line.

"Sylvia Harris on Wildwood Pegasus is the winner," the announcer bellows, and the words echo in my head as I sit up with my arms extended, my head lifted.

Peg heads toward the winner's circle like he was meant to live there. You would have thought that horse had a modeling coach, the way he posed for the photos that night in the most regal manner. On a numb sort of high, we go through the photos, the press, and the pats on the back, until it is finally time to put Peg back in his stall.

Not quite believing what has happened to both of us, I get out a handful of carrots, just like on the day we met, and Peg uses his newfound manners to only partially rip them from my hands and crunch them. I can't resist grabbing his face in my hands and breathing him in one more time. "You saved my life tonight," I tell him with tears in my eyes. I go out to greet my family, who have all come down from the stands and are moving toward me. I can see the smiles. Mioshi runs to me.

"Mommy, Mommy, you won."

I opened my arms to him—he is already at my height—and hug him as he hugs me.

"Yes. Mommy won."

It was a fairy-tale ending that cold day in December. But reality set in quickly. I rode a few more times, with mixed results, into 2008 and received a great deal of media attention. Shortly afterward I was presented with the opportunity to write my life story. I knew I couldn't give racing the focus I would need while writing a book, so I took off to write and rest. I was tired and energized at the same time—tired from training to be the best jockey I could be, and energized at the thought of telling my story hoping to be an inspiration for anyone seeking an alternate path to healing. Time off hasn't been easy.

Telling my story proved to be more frustrating than I had imagined. First, it was hard to reveal and face some truths about being me. Second, my family was still splintered and all over the globe; I was still on the search for the right medicine to level me off; and finally, I missed my horses. They were calling me back to the track, and eventually I answered. After almost a year, I returned to the sport I love.

I went back to Hawthorne Race Course, the place of my breakthrough. To my surprise, I didn't get any mounts. For the most part, I was not treated very well by many of the jockeys or people who worked with the horses in the backstretch. I picked up on an undercurrent of resentment by some who felt that I didn't deserve to be in the spotlight and others who assumed that I thought I was better than them. Nothing was further from the truth. The offer to do a book had been totally unexpected. All I really wanted to do was to ride. But I also knew the book was a chance to show how being bipolar can affect both the victims of the disorder and their families. I hope to encourage others to seek help and to know they can still lead full lives. And equally so, for me, it was a chance to pay respect to what I consider to be my lifeline—horses. My bond with them is beyond my scope of expression; they are truly my haven.

Instead of putting up a fight at Hawthorne, I decided I didn't care what people thought about me, I just wanted to ride. So I moved on to Arlington in an attempt to get mounts there. Nothing. But I learned that there might be something across the line at Indiana Downs. It was April, and if I could get on in time, I might get a chance to compete in the opening weekend, which coincided with the Kentucky Derby, making it a big weekend throughout racing. I got lucky. Now, when you're new to a track, unless you're a star, you don't get your pick of the mounts. You take what's given to you. They gave me the worst horse there, and I came in last. But I didn't care, because I was back.

The second mount proved to be more costly.

I knew something was wrong with him. After years of riding, breezing, and just loving horses, you notice these things. They could have sore muscles from working too much, have breathing problems, have bruised ankles, or hold their heads too high. This horse just wasn't right. He was broken like Peg had once been. He would lean into the rail, and I thought maybe something was wrong with his left shoulder.

I kept telling the trainer and the groom something was wrong, but they assured me that he could run the race. They said, Just let the horse break on his own and don't pull him back. I took them at their word, and the groom, under the trainer's instruction, worked on the horse's shoulder. But just in case, while in the paddock, I warned the jockey to my left that the horse liked to lean into the rail and to be aware of us down the stretch. I had a lot to prove that day, not only to the officials at the track but also to myself that I could compete again, especially after my recent last-place finish.

As soon as we jumped out of the gate, the horse to my left came up a bit, then my horse started leaning to the left. I kept giving him a little kick to steer him away from the rail, but he had decided to run the race the way he wanted. Then boom, my nightmare was about to be realized. We clipped heels with the other horse, and my horse went down. Just days before, world-class jockey Rene Douglas had fallen off a horse and sustained extensive injuries, as had another jockey, Michael Straight. Thoughts of them flashed though my head as I went sailing over the top of my horse facefirst, hard onto the track. I did not feel the pain immediately. I got up, looking for my horse. If I fall, it's very seldom I'm not still connected to the horse. Usually he's nearby, waiting for me to lead him off the track. But this one scampered away. I began to feel woozy and dropped to one knee as the medics arrived. All I could think was, Where is my horse? They told me I was fine, but

I wasn't. I had crushed the right side of my skull near the back of my neck. On my right side, four vertebrae were broken and so was my left shoulder. They carried me out on the board and straight to the hospital. It was May 4, 2009.

It would be almost a year before I could ride again.

Epilogue

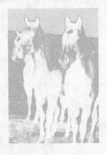

Delaware Park
Wilmington, Delaware
June 2010

I'm sitting in group therapy. This is a new experience for me. I usually shy away from discussing the challenges of being bipolar. But it's different here. I'm different here. I am constantly struck by how *nice* they are to me, especially since I was not as nice to them at first. I can't help myself at times, and when I first got here, I was too argumentative and confrontational, not caring if it cost me the chance to make friends.

For many, myself included, being bipolar makes for a lonely existence. It's caused discord with my parents, wreaked havoc on my personal relationships, and distanced me both geographically and emotionally from my three children, whom I love dearly but from afar. I have found it hard to maintain friendships for fear of what happens when my life turns into its own amusement park and I'm the star attraction. Only now have I reached out to reestablish contact with the friends with whom I grew up. It's still very difficult for me; I feel emotionally worn out by interacting with people, by the drama, by the distrust I now have. Admittedly, I haven't exhibited a great track record in establishing relationships with people that were beneficial to my well-being. I'm trying, but in truth, I feel that I would be happiest if all I had to deal with were the horses.

My journey to Wilmington began after I'd recovered from the injuries sustained in my spill at Indiana Downs. The recovery was painful. I had to wear a neck brace, and I resisted taking the pain pills prescribed by doctors because I hate medicine. I've taken so many meds over the years, I am convinced that nothing really works. So I chanted, took herbs, and did acupuncture to heal my broken body.

Unfortunately, I am part of this nation's underinsured. If you haven't figured it out yet, jockeys don't make a lot of money. They are paid per mount. The advance from the book deal helped, but, of course, I wasn't expecting an accident. I had used a good portion of the money paying off debts, getting a decent place to live, and trying to make up for time lost with my children, which featured a trip for all of us to Japan. Now, with me literally on my back, unable to ride, money became scarce.

I lived in a cute townhouse in a good neighborhood, filled with decent people, in Chicago. It had become my home, and I felt safe there. On occasion, my father would visit me with Mioshi, and it was just enough room for the three of us. Life felt good until the landlord decided to sell the townhouse, and I couldn't afford to buy it. I was forced to move out, and with little money, I really had nowhere to go. After all of the victories, I was broke, homeless once again, and not fully recovered. Still, I thought, I've been homeless before, and if I can just hold on for a few weeks, I can get back up on the horse, so to speak. Thank God, it was still summer, and it wasn't cold yet. I took what money I had left and put my things in storage. At times I even slept in my bin. During the day, I hung around Hawthorne and Arlington, willing to do anything I could, in my not fully recovered body, from feeding horses to mucking out stalls.

Having been homeless before, I knew how to navigate the streets, and with the help of the El trains, I would bide my time, riding through the city and washing up at McDonald's or at the airport, which has the best facilities for a woman in my situation. But the humiliation of having seemingly returned to a place I thought was way behind me was as difficult to deal with as anything physical.

I thought about calling my father and returning to him and Mioshi. I knew he would take me back, that now I could count on him. It's taken me years to understand that just like me, he's not perfect. But he loves me. And, more important, he loves Mioshi. There are moments when I fill up with tears when I think about how my father took on this energetic, highly creative boy and allowed him to be free. Mioshi is half black and half Latin and is full of fire. My dad loves him just the way he is, and I don't know what I would have done without him to care for my baby boy.

Still, I couldn't concede defeat. I heard there was work available at a large farm in Pennsylvania. I borrowed money from my dad and headed there; if nothing else, I would be closer to him and Mioshi. At the farm, I found work as a groom again, but not as a jockey. It was frustrating, and I was still in pain from my accident and took to drinking beer to ease it, or maybe just to fill the boredom.

It was coming up on a year since my accident and I missed the action of the racetrack. After a month in Pennsylvania, I headed to Charlestown, West Virginia, to see if I could get some mounts at the track there. It was here that I began to see the changes taking place in the American economy now creeping into the racing game. Suddenly, the big-name jockeys were taking mounts they would've passed up at one time. As a consequence, there were fewer mounts available, which made it harder for a rider like me, trying to make a comeback. Again, I could only find work as a groom, that and trouble.

I started drinking more than beer. Drinking is a trigger for me and I should stay away from it. But I didn't. It is particularly difficult to do if you're staying on the backstretch. The horse industry seems to lure troubled people. The lifestyle is transient and few questions are asked; you can drink and drug without much provocation, until somebody tells on you or you get sloppy and it shows. I was getting sloppy with it. I was drinking, and to fit in, I was starting to hang out with the wrong types; I even began dabbling with drugs. I realized I needed to get out of there, and, although it was a struggle, I left for Wilmington. Someone had told me about Delaware Park and how it was known for its support programs for the many broken lives of those connected to the racing world.

When I got to Delaware Park, one of the more prestigious racetracks in the country, I met Charles, a worker on the backstretch. He saw me sitting in the Horseman's Lounge, where some racetrack business is conducted and information regarding the horses and races are posted. We started talking and he took pity on me. He signed for me to get onto the backside, which enabled me to talk to trainers and look for work. He even let me stay in his room at the dormitory, eventually having to kick me out because of my behavior. He told me about a counselor there, Wesley Jones, who might be able to help me. I was skeptical; every track has a psychologist or abuse counselors who work with you, but they often work *against* you by not trying to help those on the backstretch to get to the core of their problems. Still, I knew I should go; I was starting to drown again.

Wesley looked at my file and said that he'd never seen a case like mine. In addition to being bipolar, he is certain that I have anger management issues coupled with substance abuse because of my father's alcoholism. I explained that I had tried drugs in the past, but that wasn't my primary problem. I'm a drinker. But he differed, saying that life on the backstretch for someone like me could easily lead to drug abuse, and he wanted to prevent the worst from happening.

Wesley found me a doctor who actually listened to me and my concerns about medication. She prescribed Zyprexa, which has had minimal side effects. I've never wanted to risk riding while on medication. A groggy, less-than-focused jockey is asking for trouble. But here at Delaware Park, they care more about me as a person than the consequences of me being in a manic state while riding. They insist on me sticking with my medications. I can't pursue my career unless I can show that I am doing everything I can to combat my demons. That means I cannot skip taking my medicine, or any counseling that is necessary to keep me functional.

And I'm actually enjoying group and anger management therapy. I've learned that there are people who are just like me and even worse. I'll never be cured, but the condition can be managed, if I'm willing. At forty-three, I'm willing. If I can't get my act together, I will be forced out of the track world and away from the one thing that means the most to me: the horses.

My life is simple in Wilmington. I've learned that a routine is important for someone like me. I work out, go to group, see my doctor, breeze and gallop horses, or bale hay and feed my equine friends. When I can get mounts, I race with the hope of winning. I recently came in first while here at Delaware Park, and I'm proud of that. I'm starting to get more mounts.

But I have a long way to go. I'm trying to stop my running from one place to the next. The problems always follow like a shadow. At least here, at Delaware Park, I have been forced to see and accept the patient compassion and help of others and to realize that my life is in my hands.

I'm an apprentice jockey. Soon I will have enough mounts to qualify as a journeyman jockey, which allows for the best horses and top money. I believe I still have time to realize my biggest dream: to race in the Kentucky Derby. After that, I'd like to hang up my silks and become a trainer. There are very few African American trainers, and I would like to join that auspicious group.

I also want to be a better mother and daughter.

The relationship I've had with my children has been tough. My two oldest have been through a lot. Shauna, almost twenty, is a beautiful blend of her father and me. She lives in London, where she's going to college and working as a waitress. There's a distance between us that, in time, I hope will shorten as we grow to love and respect each other even more.

Ryan is complicated. The middle child, he probably needs me the most, but will never admit it. We often clash. I don't know why, we just do. He just graduated from high school.

And then there's Mioshi. We clash too, but it's fun. Mioshi is my love child. Although briefly, his father touched me in a way I haven't experienced with another man. I hope that Mioshi knows that he was, for me, conceived in love. He's vibrant, alive, and possesses an in-your-face creative flair that I admire and envy. He's strong, maybe the strongest of my children. My dad has given him a steady foundation, and for half of his life it was me and him against the world.

Oh, how I long for the days when it was just me and my three Musketeers. When I could, I was very hands-on with my children. We did arts and crafts, went to the park, the library, and the beach. And we were happy in our own little world where Mommy is wild and fun. But the fun would often come to an end when my problems surfaced and parents, friends, and social workers had to intervene, forcing a calm that used to make me ache. I know now that it was necessary, but it still doesn't erase the hurt.

And then there's my mom. For years I thought that she didn't understand me. We don't get along. I know now that she was overwhelmed and didn't quite know what to do with me. One night her sweet daughter went to bed; before dawn she was up screaming at imaginary acid rain and frogs falling from the sky. It must have been terrifying for her, because she couldn't make it better. That's what moms want to do. We want to make it better, even when we can't.

My relationship with my mother is fragile, partly because her illness has taken its toll. I almost lost her recently, as her Crohn's disease worsened. I found out about it when my children announced they were coming to the United States but heading straight to California to see their grandmother and not visiting me. After badgering them for an answer, I learned that my mother was very ill, and it was as if they were coming home to say good-bye.

After I learned that my entire family was going to California to say good-bye to Mom, I found my way to California. This was before I was homeless again, and I had just enough money to buy a ticket and rush to her side. When I showed up in her room, she looked at me and said sarcastically, "What are you doing here?" That may sound rough but it's become a coping mechanism for Mom, who's walked with me through many a nightmare.

I looked at her frail body and realized that if something were to happen to this woman, I would be devastated. She's my mom and I love her and I'm sorry. Sorry for the worry and the wreckage I have left behind for her to clean up at times. Sorry that I couldn't be the perfect daughter she wanted me to be. And yet I know she doesn't want or need an apology from me. That's why when I saw her in that bed, I did what any girl would do with her mom. I crawled in bed with her. I wanted to feel her heart beat and know she was still alive. That she is still here for me.

There's no cure for bipolar disorder. There are medicines and theories and studies and nut houses. None of those things work for me. The horses keep me sane and alive more than anything. As long as I have my family, broken or not, and the horses I will survive.

Will I make it? I don't know. I'm a long shot. But someday, I'll be a winner, and I'm learning you don't always have to come in first to accomplish that.

Acknowledgments

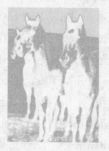

I would like to express my sincere and heartfelt gratitude to everyone who helped bring this book to life and to all of you holding it now for letting my life be a part of yours—if only for a moment.

Mom and Dad, U.S. Army veterans: I love and thank you for everything you gave to me as a little girl, for shaping my life and the lives of my children, for loving me even in silence, separation, and confusion, and for allowing me to be a full-grown brat to this day. I appreciate your troubles and hardship. To my children: Thank you for being beautiful and strong, for giving me something to be proud of, for going on, no matter what, and for giving me a reason to go on too, when I had all but given up. I appreciate you all and everyone who has taken care of you when I wasn't able, nurturing you in the midst of a torn family. I give my sincere thanks to Nichiren Daishonin's Buddhism for giving me a foundation of faith even when I felt unworthy. To all the wonderful, wise, and healing horses, mentors, and friends—those of you who helped me to believe in myself and be a winner the way we are all meant to be.

Thank you, Judy Smith, for rescuing me from my destructive self and becoming a best friend. I needed a compassionate one who would never turn away. You proved to me again what it means to be a humanist in daily life. Elyse Cheney, my literary agent: We made it! Thank you for letting me grow throughout this process and for showing me a side of tenacity I hadn't known. Eunetta Boone and William Boulware, coauthors, how you worked your magic is beyond words. My gratefulness to you, I hope, is fully understood. I am proud and touched by your dedication and thoughtfulness. Thank you both tremendously for making this happen with no thought of self first. Dawn Davis, HarperCollins editor extraordinaire, thank you for not giving up on this project when I definitely had walked away. Your faith is deeply appreciated.

Wesley Jones and the Backstretch Employee Assistance Program at Delaware Park, I will always be appreciative of the backbone you made me find again and the boundaries you taught me to set. Again, you saved my life. I would also like to thank every person for being who they are and for somehow, no matter what, triumphing in life and spirit. I want to encourage you all to find or continue to follow a dream, a wish, an ambition. Overcome the obstacles, never give up, and thank the story that is your life. It's your show; you are the star. Last of all I want to thank my bipolar life and the horses that saved me.